Raymond T. Krediet
Dirk G. Struijk
Sadie van Esch

Peritoneal Dialysis Manual

A Guide for Understanding the Treatment

5 figures and 6 tables, 2018

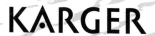

Basel · Freiburg · Paris · London · New York ·
Chennai · New Delhi · Bangkok · Beijing · Shanghai ·
Tokyo · Kuala Lumpur · Singapore · Sydney

Raymond T. Krediet, MD, PhD

Professor of Nephrology

Division of Nephrology, Department of Medicine

Academic Medical Center

P.O. Box 22700

NL–1100 DE Amsterdam (The Netherlands)

Library of Congress Cataloging-in-Publication Data

Names: Krediet, R. T., author. | Struijk, D. G., author. | Esch, Sadie van., author.
Title: Peritoneal dialysis manual : a guide for understanding the treatment / Raymond T. Krediet, Dirk G. Struijk, Sadie van Esch.
Description: Basel ; New York : Karger, 2018. | Includes bibliographical references and index.
Identifiers: LCCN 2018015734| ISBN 9783318063790 (soft cover : alk. paper) | ISBN 9783318063806 (electronic version)
Subjects: | MESH: Peritoneal Dialysis
Classification: LCC RC901.7.P48 | NLM WJ 378 | DDC 617.4/61059--dc23 LC record available at https://lccn.loc.gov/2018015734

Drug Dosage

The authors and the publisher have exerted every effort to ensure that drug selection and dosage set forth in this text are in accord with current recommendations and practice at the time of publication. However, in view of ongoing research, changes in government regulations, and the constant flow of information relating to drug therapy and drug reactions, the reader is urged to check the package insert for each drug for any change in indications and dosage and for added warnings and precautions. This is particularly important when the recommended agent is a new and/or infrequently employed drug.

© Copyright 2018 by S. Karger AG, P.O. Box, CH–4009 Basel (Switzerland)
www.karger.com
Printed on acid-free and non-aging paper (ISO 9706)
ISBN 978–3–318–06379–0
eISBN 978–3–318–06380–6

Contents

Foreword

During the 40 years of my career in academic nephrology, there were many opportunities and occasions for meeting and establishing long-time friendships with many colleagues in nephrology. In particular during my tenure as Editor-in-Chief of *Nephrology Dialysis Transplantation* and Chair of the International Society of Nephrology (ISN) Continuing Medical Education Program, I was and still am so fortunate to be part of this global nephrological community. Outstanding among these relationships is the long-term and highly esteemed friendship with Prof. em. Raymond "Ray" Krediet of the Academic Medical Center, University of Amsterdam.

My first "official" meeting with Ray was somewhat "uneasy" because I was invited by the Faculty of Medicine of the University of Amsterdam to be the "extra muros" jury member of Ray's PhD thesis, which was devoted to one of the first in-depth pathophysiological investigations on peritoneal transport and its various clinical aspects. Since it is expected from an "extra muros" opponent jury member to ask at least one or two intelligent questions during the public defense, I remember my great difficulty in formulating these questions because Ray's work was already at that time (1986) thorough, original, and reflected highly intelligent planning. Since then I have increasingly admired the logical continuation of the peritoneal dialysis (PD) research program by many brilliant young collaborators inspired and supervised by Ray during all the subsequent years. In this way, an internationally recognized and highly esteemed "true PD school" has established in Amsterdam.

Our understanding of the anatomy and physiology of the peritoneal membrane has tremendously increased over the years, and the advantages of PD in the overall management of end-stage kidney diseases became better realized. It became clear that the patient outcomes are comparable to and more cost-effective than those with hemodialysis. These benefits have, however, not led to increased PD utilization. Although PD is a valid renal replacement therapy when incorporated in an overall integrated care program for the patient suffering from end-stage renal disease, it has not yet established as a true long-term dialysis modality. The variable trends in PD use reflect the multiple challenges in prescribing this therapy to patients, and although its use is increasing in some countries, including China, the USA and Thailand, it has proportionally decreased in parts of Europe and Japan. Key strategies for facilitating PD utilization include the implementation of policies and incentives that favor this modality, enabling the appropriate production and supply of PD fluid at a low cost, and, very importantly, appropriate training for nephrologists and other renal care providers. I believe that in addition to the training of nephrologists, greater efforts should be made to improve the basic knowledge of PD in other medical fields, including general practices and other nonnephrological health care. Very often the patient in need of initiating dialysis will seek advice from his general practitioner or family doctor, a renal nurse, or a social worker on the different modalities of renal replacement therapy. Indeed, nurses play a vital role in patient choices by providing accurate information backed up by world-class research to patients about the potential benefits of PD. Lack of familiarity with PD of these health care providers unavoidably leads to biased advice to their patients. It is believed that part of the gap between the desired and the observed modality mix of renal replacement therapies, for example in Europe, may be due to suboptimal information provision to patients, and patient surveys have revealed that there is an association between the involvement in modality selection and patient satisfaction.

The present booklet, entitled *Peritoneal Dialysis Manual: A Guide for Understanding the Treatment*, written by *Ray T. Krediet, Dirk G. Struijk,* and *Sadie van Esch,* meets the need for a practical handbook offering sensible advice but also detailed information on virtually all clinical and pathophysiological aspects of PD in a readily accessible format. The easy, small format should fit in a white coat pocket of a nephrologist or resident in nephrology and internal medicine seeing a PD patient during rounds or in the outpatient ambulatory setting. This book should, however, also be of relevance, use, and interest to all other health care workers involved in the treatment of patients suffering from end-stage renal disease – nurses, pharmacists, dieticians, intensivists, and medical students. The fact that the majority of the chapters are written by a single author able to explain the complexities of PD in a clear but still scientific and comprehensive way is one of the attractive aspects of this work. I recommend this booklet since I am convinced that it is an excellent addition to the PD library in every renal unit worldwide.

Norbert Lameire, MD, PhD
Emeritus Professor of Medicine and Nephrology
Medical Faculty of the University of Ghent, Belgium

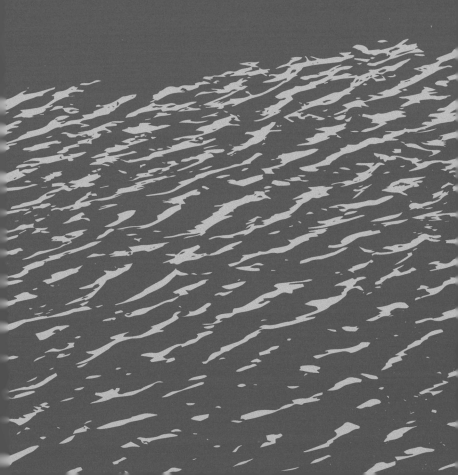

Chapter 1

Anatomy and Physiology of the Peritoneum

Anatomy and Physiology of the Peritoneum

The peritoneum, which can be used as a dialysis membrane, consists of the mesothelium and the underlying interstitial tissue that contains the microvessels. In adults, the mesothelial surface area averages at 0.55 m² by CT scanning, which is about one third of the skin surface. Solutes and water are transported from peritoneal capillaries through the interstitium and mesothelium to the dialysate-filled peritoneal cavity and vice versa. The mesothelium offers no resistance to transport; the possible role of the interstitium will be discussed later.

Solute Transport

The number of peritoneal capillaries perfused is the most important determinant of solute transport, not the peritoneal blood flow. Endothelial transport occurs through an abundance of transendothelial pores and interendothelial water channels. Small solutes like urea, creatinine, and glucose traverse the endothelium by diffusion through small pores that have radii of about 40 Å. Even β_2-microglobulin, which has a radius of 17 Å, can pass the small pores without hindrance. Consequently, the differences in the transport of various small solutes are dependent on differences in their diffusion velocity (molecular weight [MW] and shape) and not on the intrinsic permeability of the peritoneal membrane. The transperitoneal concentration gradient of a solute is the 3rd determinant of diffusion. It decreases during a dialysis dwell due to saturation of the dialysate. Consequently, the dialysate/plasma ratio, which equals 0 in the beginning of a dialysis exchange, increases during the dwell and

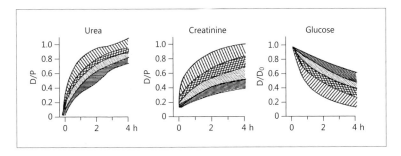

Fig. 1. The various solute transport categories. Note that the high creatinine transporters have the fastest disappearance of glucose. D/P, dialysate/plasma concentration ratio; D/D_0, dialysate concentration at a time/dialysate concentration before inflow.

finally reaches 1.0, at which time no effective diffusion occurs. For urea (MW 60 Da), this equilibrium is approached after 4 h in many patients. In this situation, the drained dialysate volume is the only determinant for the removal of urea from the body. Equilibrium for creatinine (MW 113 Da) takes longer. Diffusion also occurs for intraperitoneally administered osmotic agents like glucose (MW 180 Da). The absorption of glucose averages 60% after 4 h, which has a marked effect on its osmotic activity during a dwell.

Marked differences in peritoneal solute transport are present among patients, dependent on the magnitude of the effective surface area and thus the number of microvessels perfused. The dialysate/plasma ratio of creatinine after a dwell time of 4 h can range between 0.34 and 1.00 (mean 0.65). Based on mean values and standard deviations of a stable peritoneal dialysis (PD) population, patients have been divided into high, low, and average (high and low average) transporters, as shown in Figure 1.

The above terminology is very confusing, because high transporters usually have low ultrafiltration (UF) rates, caused by a high glucose absorption, which leads to a rapid disappearance of the osmotic gradient. A low ultrafiltered volume results in impaired removal of urea and other small molecules. Because of this phenomenon "high" is better replaced by "fast" and "low" by "slow." Fast transporters have an increased risk of overhydration. A meta-analysis reported that patients with a fast transport status had higher mortality than the others. However, this was only the case for those treated with CAPD (continuous ambulatory PD) and glucose as osmotic agent. The CAPD scheme consists of 3 short dwells (4–6 h) and 1 long dwell (8–10 h). Especially during the long dwell, fluid removal can be low or absent. Fast-transport patients treated with APD (automated PD) in whom a long dwell can be avoided had no increased mortality. Survival was also not impaired in patients treated with icodextrin (a poorly absorbed high-MW osmotic agent) for the long dwell. Long-term PD is often associated with the development of fast small-solute transport rates, pointing to a large effective surface area due to diabetiform neoangiogenesis. A fast transport status can also occur early in the time course of PD, for instance in patients with inflammation due to marked vascular comorbidity as well as by the development of endothelial-mesenchymal transition (EMT) of mesothelial cells. Clinically, this is characterized by fast solute transport, high effluent concentrations of the mesothelial cell marker cancer antigen (CA)-125, and also by high effluent levels of the vascular endothelial growth factor. The latter is an important mediator of diabetic retinopathy. Some have claimed that EMT is an early stage of long-term structural peritoneal abnormalities but without proof. The functional changes of EMT in PD are a transitory phenomenon.

Table 1. Pressure gradients

	In dialysate filled peritoneal cavity	Pressure gradient
Hydrostatic pressure, mm Hg	8 (recumbent)	17
Colloid osmotic pressure, mm Hg	0.1	−21
Osmolality, mosm/kg H_2O	347 (glucose 1.36%) 486 (glucose 3.86%)	Dependent on the RC
Initial crystalloid osmotic pressure gradient, mm Hg for RC = 0.03	Glucose 1.36% Glucose 3.86%	24 105
RC, reflection coefficient.		

Fluid Transport

Removal of excess fluid from the body is probably the most important goal of PD. The transport of water and dissolved solutes to and from the peritoneal cavity is determined by hydrostatic and osmotic pressure gradients and also by lymphatic drainage. The pressure gradients that influence transcapillary UF are summarized in Table 1. The effectiveness of the crystalloid osmotic pressure is determined by the osmolality of the solution and its capability to induce a pressure gradient across a membrane. The latter is dependent on the reflection coefficient. This parameter can range between 0 and 1.0. The solute passes the membrane without any hindrance and has no osmotic effect when 0. A reflection coefficient of 1.0 means that the membrane is semipermeable, i.e., that the solute cannot pass, but water can. In this situation, 1 mosm/kg H_2O induces an osmotic pressure of 19.3 mm Hg. The reflection coefficient of glucose across the peritoneum averages at 0.03, meaning that large osmolality gradients are required to induce a crystalloid osmotic pressure gradient. These gradients decrease during a dwell due to absorption of glucose. The glucose absorption explains why the intraperitoneal volume increases initially and decreases thereafter.

Replacement of glucose by the glucose polymer icodextrin (see Chapter 9 Peritoneal Dialysis Solutions) causes sustained UF, because it hardly diffuses from the peritoneal cavity and creates a colloid osmotic pressure gradient.

The paradoxical observation that glucose causes UF despite its low reflection coefficient is explained by the presence of the water channel aquaporin-1 (AQP-1) in capillary and venular peritoneal endothelial cells. Solutes cannot traverse AQP-1, meaning that the reflection coefficient of glucose to this channel equals 1.0. Therefore, AQP-1 induces free water transport (FWT). The initial contribution of FWT to total transcapillary UF averages 40%. FWT explains the decrease in dialysate Na^+ (sodium sieving), a dilutional phenomenon that occurs in the initial phase of a dwell with the highest glucose concentration. Icodextrin only induces fluid transport through the small pores and thus no sodium sieving.

Assessment of lymphatic absorption from the peritoneal cavity and tissues requires the use of a macromolecular marker, where diffusion can be neglected. The marker can be given intravenously or intraperitoneally. In the first case, the appearance rate in the dialysate is measured, and in the other case the disappearance rate from the dialysate. The values obtained with the appearance rates average 0.2 mL/min, those with the disappearance rate 1.5 mL/min. The difference can partly be explained by the absence of a steady state for the appearance rate and by transmesothelial transport of the intraperitoneal marker to the interstitium. Clinical research has mainly been done using the peritoneal clearance (disappearance rate) of neutral dextran. Consequently, the method gives an assessment of overall lymphatic uptake, i.e., from the peritoneal cavity and from the interstitial tissues. Results of those studies showed that the effective lymphatic absorption rate is influenced by the intraperitoneal pressure but hardly by posture. Also, the duration of PD has no effect. A small minority of patients have a high value already in the beginning of PD. These patients often have otherwise unexplained UF failure (UFF).

UFF is by far the most important complication of long-term PD, because it often leads to overhydration. The two must clearly be distinguished, because overhydration can also develop because of a decrease in residual urine production, excessive fluid intake, an inadequate dialysis prescription, or peritoneal leakage. Therefore, the diagnosis UFF should be based on a standardized dialysis exchange. According to the 3 × 4 rule, UFF is present when net UF after a 4-h dwell is <400 mL using a dialysis solution based on 3.86%/4.25% glucose. Early UFF is often not a big risk for overhydration, because most patients will still have urine production. Acute peritonitis causes temporary UFF, because the effective peritoneal surface area is enlarged due to the effect of inflammation on the number of peritoneal microvessels perfused, which leads to a rapid disappearance of the crystalloid osmotic gradient. Late UFF is a serious complication, because it is associated with structural peritoneal abnormalities and often leads to overhydration. Late UFF is present in about 20% of patients treated with PD for >2 years. Enlargement of the vascular peritoneal surface area is the most frequent cause, because it leads to a rapid disappearance of the crystalloid osmotic pressure gradient. Long-term exposure to the extremely high glucose concentrations in the dialysis solutions causes diabetiform neoangiogenesis and vasculopathy. The latter is likely to reduce the filtration pressure and thereby ultrafiltration. A decreased osmotic conductance of glucose may develop during long-term PD and also cause UFF. This reduced sensitivity of glucose to induce UF can be explained by a decrease in FWT, as evidenced by a declined sodium sieving. AQP-1 damage or dysfunction is probably not the cause, a more likely explanation is the binding of filtered water in fibrotic peritoneal interstitial tissue, because collagen binds water. This is supported by the extremely reduced sodium sieving that is present in patients with encapsulating peritoneal sclerosis.

Suggested Reading

Heimburger O, Waniewski J, Werynski A, Lindholm B:
A quantitative description of solute and fluid transport during peritoneal dialysis.
Kidney Int 1992;41:1320–1332.

Krediet RT, Lindholm B, Rippe B:
Pathophysiology of peritoneal membrane failure.
Perit Dial Int 2000;20(suppl 4):S22–S42.

Krediet RT:
Peritoneal dialysis: from bench to bedside.
Clin Kidney J 2013;6:568–577.

Nolph KD, Twardowski ZJ, Popovich RP, Rubin J:
Equilibration of peritoneal dialysis solutions during long-dwell exchanges.
J Lab Clin Med 1979;93:246–256.

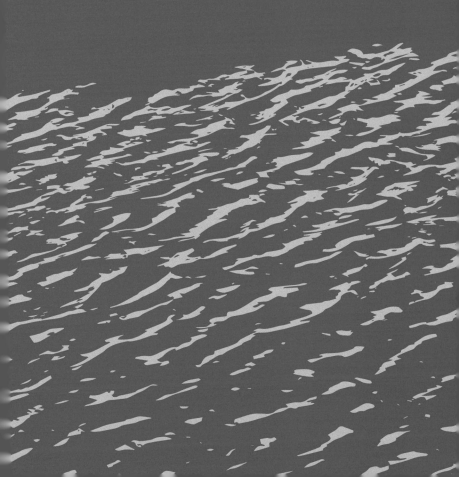

Chapter 2
Treatment Modalities

Treatment Modalities

Treatment Choice

Peritoneal dialysis (PD) can be performed either manually (continuous ambulatory PD [CAPD]) or by using a cycler (automated PD [APD]). Both treatments are equal in terms of clinical outcome. When choosing between both techniques, patient preferences play a major role. With CAPD, treatment is largely performed during the day. This is in contrast to the treatment with APD, which mainly takes place in the late evening and at night. CAPD, therefore, interferes more than APD with the daily schedule, which, for example, can be an impediment to having a full-time job or other daily activities. In addition to the psychosocial aspects, there are also medical indications that can play a role in the choice between CAPD and APD. These indications can be divided into 2 categories, namely improving the dialysis adequacy and lowering the intraperitoneal pressure. The first category consists mainly of patients with a rapid loss of osmotic gradient in the dialysate due to rapid resorption, which makes frequent changes with a short residence time useful. The second category comprises patients who suffer from lack of space in the abdominal cavity. For example, patients with polycystic kidney disease often suffer from hernias or recurrence of dialysate leakage. APD enables this patient group to perform frequent changes with a smaller inflow volume. In addition, intraperitoneal pressure is also lowest in the supine position.

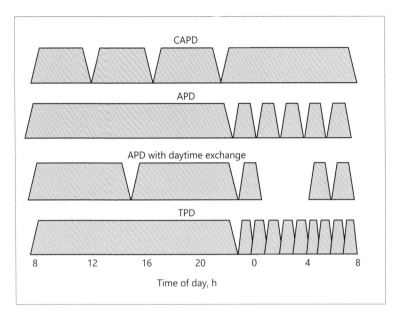

Fig. 1. The various peritoneal dialysis (PD) schemes. APD, automated PD; CAPD, continuous ambulatory PD; TPD, tidal PD.

Continuous Ambulatory Peritoneal Dialysis

The prescription of PD in CAPD is straightforward. The manual exchanges usually take 30–60 min and are performed 3–5 times a day (Fig. 1). Because of the long dwells, only the total volume drained (not peritoneal membrane characteristics) are relevant for dialysate adequacy.

Incremental PD can be considered when sufficient residual renal function is present. This implies that the dialysis dose is gradually extended on the basis of the declining residual renal function.

This might consist of only 1 exchange with 1.5–2 L of glucose containing dialysate or icodextrin, depending on the need for ultrafiltration. In time, the dialysis dose can be increased by increasing the exchange frequency or the dwell volume. Increasing the dwell volume first – and thereby decreasing the number of dwells – is advantageous for the patient with respect to the treatment burden, and it is also cost-effective. Measuring the intraperitoneal pressure can be of help in determining the optimal intraperitoneal volume.

When a glucose-sparing regimen is followed, one of the short dwells with glucose can be replaced by an amino acid-containing solution. When more ultrafiltration is needed, to avoid high glucose concentrations, icodextrin should be introduced for the longest dwell first. However, the value of glucose-sparing strategies for the preservation of the peritoneal membrane has currently not been demonstrated in clinical trials.

To increase the dialysis dose, the only available options are increasing the volume to the maximum the patient can tolerate (taking the impact on net ultrafiltration into account) and increasing the number of exchanges to 5 per day.

Automated Peritoneal Dialysis

The prescription of APD is more complex than CAPD as many variables can be modified, and patient characteristics can also be taken into account. While in CAPD saturation of the effluent with low-molecular-weight particles has usually occurred due to the long residence time of the dialysate in the abdomen, this is not the case during the shorter dwells in APD. Especially in patients with a slow transport from the blood to the dialysate in the peritoneal cavity, this can lead to inadequate dialysis.

The initial prescription of APD usually consists of a nightly treatment of 8 or 9 h combined with 1 long daily dwell. During the night, 3–4 exchanges are performed by the cycler. To increase the dialysis dose, like in CAPD, usually the first step is to optimize the dialysate volume, which can be accomplished more gradually. The next step depends both on patient preference and membrane characteristics. In most cases, adding an additional daily exchange, either manually or cycler driven, is the best option. Alternatively, the nightly treatment time can be prolonged for a few hours to 10–12 h. The last option is to increase the number of exchanges during night to maximally 6 or 7, but this is only effective in patients with a fast transport.

In contrast to CAPD, patients performing APD are at risk of inadequate sodium removal, as this mainly takes place by connective sodium transport. This is caused by sodium sieving when using short dwells. However, this deficit can be compensated by using icodextrin for the long daily dwell.

Tidal Automated Peritoneal Dialysis

Tidal dialysis is a special form of APD. In contrast to APD, in which the dialysate is completely drained at the end of the cycle, during tidal APD only part of the dialysate is drained before the start of a new cycle (Fig. 1). The percentage of the inflow volume that is not drained is usually 50–75%. This treatment mode does not improve solute clearances and fluid removal as compared to conventional non-tidal APD. However, it can be helpful in reducing abdominal discomfort and nightly alarms during the treatment in case of catheter outflow problems or abdominal complaints during complete drainage. When setting the cycler, it must be indicated how much has to be withdrawn during the treatment. If this is misjudged, the possibility exists that the intraperitoneal volume at the end of the cycles differs greatly from the original inflow volume.

Suggested Reading

Dejardin A, Robert A, Goffin E:
Intraperitoneal pressure in PD patients: relationship to intraperitoneal volume, body size and PD-related complications.
Nephrol Dial Transplant 2007;22:1437–1444.

Perez RA, Blake PG, McMurray S, Mupas L, Oreopoulos DG:
What is the optimal frequency of cycling in automated peritoneal dialysis?
Perit Dial Int 2000;20:548–556.

Rabindranath KS, Adams J, Ali TZ, MacLeod AM, Vale L, Cody JD, Wallace SA, Daly C:
Continuous ambulatory peritoneal dialysis versus automated peritoneal dialysis for end-stage renal disease.
Cochrane Database Sys Rev 2007;2:CD006515.

Rodríguez-Carmona A, Fontán MP:
Sodium removal in patients undergoing CAPD and automated peritoneal dialysis.
Perit Dial Int 2002;22:705–713.

Struijk DG:
Dosing of peritoneal dialysis;
in Magee CC, Tucker JK, Singh AK (eds):
Core Concepts in Dialysis and Continuous Therapies.
Dordrecht, Springer, 2016, pp 113–120.

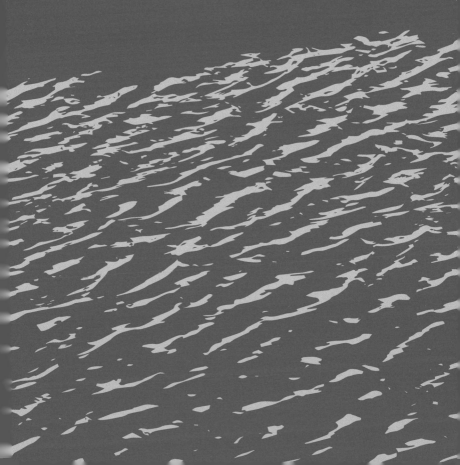

Chapter 3

Access- and Catheter-Related Complications

Access- and Catheter-Related Complications

Peritoneal Dialysis Catheters

Permanent access to the abdominal cavity is essential for the treatment with peritoneal dialysis. Probably the most commonly used catheter was developed by Tenckhoff and Schlechter in 1968. This catheter has a straight configuration and possesses 1 or 2 Dacron cuffs for anchorage to the abdominal wall. Later, catheters were developed with a U-shaped configuration in the abdominal wall (swan neck catheters) resulting in an exit site that was directed downwards. Also, catheters have been made with intraperitoneal configurations ending in curls or a weighted tip. However, comparative studies between the different catheters are scarce and often of poor quality. No single catheter has been demonstrated to be superior to all others. A recent meta-analysis concluded that catheters with a straight intraperitoneal segment had the best survival.

Implantation Techniques

The majority of peritoneal dialysis catheters are inserted using the open surgical technique. Alternative procedures are (advanced) laparoscopic implantation and percutaneous techniques. Since no good evidence exists that any of these procedures is superior to the others, local expertise at individual centers by dedicated teams should govern the choice of the method for catheter insertion. Subcutaneous burying of the catheter until use, which was promoted by Moncrief et al. [1993], may have advantages for the association between the timing of catheter insertion and the beginning of dialysis. According to the International Society for Peritoneal Dialysis (ISPD), >80% of catheters should be patent at 1 year when censored for death or elective modality change.

Timing of Catheter Implantation in Relation to the Start of Dialysis

It is recommended to plan the catheter insertion timely in order to enable a healing time of 2 weeks before starting dialysis. This will reduce early dialysate leakage. In urgent starters, it is advised to reduce the intraperitoneal pressure by using smaller dialysate volumes in the supine position to reduce early leakage.

Preoperative Preparations

In addition to the routine screening for an operation, special attention must be paid to assessing the abdomen with respect to the presence of scars, hernias, and space-occupying organs such as polycystic kidneys. Preparation of the bowel with laxatives is advised, and the bladder should be emptied before the procedure. The location of the exit site should be marked in advance in a sitting or standing position. Whether screening for methicillin-resistant *Staphylococcus aureus* (MRSA) and nasal carriage of *S. aureus* is warranted depends on their occurrence and local expertise. Although the evidence is limited, antibiotic prophylaxis is advised during the catheter implantation procedure.

Postoperative Care

Until healing, usually the first 5–6 weeks, the exit site should be covered by a sterile and nonocclusive bandage. During that time, the bandage should be changed by a nurse using a sterile technique. In order to promote the healing and ingrowth of the cuffs, it is necessary to fix the catheter properly. After healing, the patient can take over exit site care according to the local protocol. Although current practice can vary per center, in most centers the abdomen is flushed after implantation in order to remove remaining blood. Thereafter, the catheter is flushed once every 1–2 weeks until the start of dialysis to prevent obstruction.

Catheter-Related Complications

Postoperative Complications

Hemorrhage, perforation of bladder or bowels, exit site leakage and infection, and catheter dysfunction are postoperative complications that can occur after implantation. According to the ISPD, the frequency of these complications should be monitored. Perforation and significant hemorrhage should be <1% and postoperative leakage <5%. The treatment of these complications is described in Chapter 6 Peritonitis and Other Catheter-Related Infections.

Late Catheter-Related Complications
(Exit Site Infections Excluded)

Leakage
Exit Site Leakage
Leakage of intraabdominal dialysate through the exit site may occur early as well as late in the treatment of PD. It is sometimes associated with an exit site infection or increased intraperitoneal pressure for instance by increasing the intraperitoneal volume or by coughing. The diagnosis is easily made by demonstration of a high glucose concentration in the fluid. It can be treated by interrupting the dialysis for 2 weeks. In case of recurrence, reducing the intraperitoneal volume and thereby reducing the intraperitoneal pressure can help. If this is not successful, replacement of the catheter might be necessary.

Pericatheter Leaks
Leakage of dialysate can also occur into the abdominal wall. These leaks can go unnoticed and only express themselves as a loss of ultrafiltration and/or weight gain. Also, edema around the exit site or implantation scar without pedal edema can occur. These leaks can be confirmed with radiological or nuclear techniques by adding contrast or technetium-99m to the dialysate. The treatment is equal to that of exit site leaks.

Catheter Migration
Ideally, the tip of the catheter should be positioned within the pelvis. However, also catheters with their tip outside the pelvis can function well. When the patient presents himself with outflow problems, the position of the catheter can be verified by a plain abdominal X-ray and, when available, compared with the position in earlier images.

The initial treatment is to prescribe laxative drugs. If this is not successful, an intervention radiologist is sometimes able to reposition the catheter by using a guidewire or Fogarty balloon. A stiff wire using the whiplash technique is not possible in swan neck catheters. The risk of another catheter dislocation is increased after successful repositioning. When the intervention is not successful, laparoscopic repositioning or replacement of the catheter by the surgeon are the final options.

Obstruction

One-way obstruction, resulting in reduced outflow, can be caused by catheter migration (as described earlier) but also by intraperitoneal adhesions resulting in pocket formation, partial occlusion of the catheter holes by fibrin, or by omental wrapping. The inflow can be tested using a 50-cm^3 syringe. If fibrin is present in the effluent, thrombolytics, e.g., tissue plasmin activator or urokinase, can be used in an attempt to dissolve the fibrin deposits. The diagnosis can be made by contrast inflow under fluoroscopic guidance. Pocket formation and omental wrapping usually require surgical intervention. Two-way obstruction is less frequent than one-way obstruction. The causes for the obstruction are identical, imaging is limited to a plain X-ray, and the obstruction mostly results in surgical intervention.

Hernias

The overall prevalence of hernias is reported to be about 10%. Hernias at the implantation site are less frequent. Reducing the dwell volume can help to avoid surgery. When surgery is unavoidable, the dialysis treatment should be interrupted for 4–6 weeks when possible. If not, smaller inflow volumes and or dialysis in the supine position should be performed.

Organ Erosion

Erosion of an organ by the catheter, mostly the bowels, is a rare event and is usually diagnosed by the occurrence of a peritonitis episode with multiple microorganisms, at least after a perforation. The treatment is removal of the catheter and correction of the perforation.

Suggested Reading

Crabtree JH:
Peritoneal dialysis catheter implantation: avoiding problems
and optimizing outcomes.
Semin Dial 2015;28:12–15.

Figueiredo A, Goh BL, Jenkins S, Johnson DW, Mactier R, Ramalakshmi S,
Shrestha B, Struijk D, Wilkie M; International Society for Peritoneal Dialysis:
Clinical practice guidelines for peritoneal access.
Perit Dial Int 2010;30:424–429.

Hagen SM, Lafranca JA, IJzermans JN, Dor FJ:
A systematic review and meta-analysis of the influence of peritoneal
dialysis catheter type on complication rate and catheter survival.
Kidney Int 2014;85:920–932.

Moncrief JW, Popovich RP, Broadrick LJ, He ZZ, Simmons EE, Tate RA:
The Moncrief-Popovich catheter. A new peritoneal access technique for
patients on peritoneal dialysis.
ASAIO J 1993;39:62–65.

Strippoli GFM, Tong A, Johnson DW, Schena FP, Craig JC:
Catheter type, placement and insertion techniques for preventing peritonitis in
peritoneal dialysis patients.
Cochrane Database Syst Rev 2004;4:CD004680.

Stuart S, Booth TC, Cash CJ, Hameeduddin A, Goode JA, Harvey C, Malhotra A:
Complications of continuous ambulatory peritoneal dialysis.
Radiographics 2009;29:441–460.

Chapter 4

Measurement of Peritoneal Transport

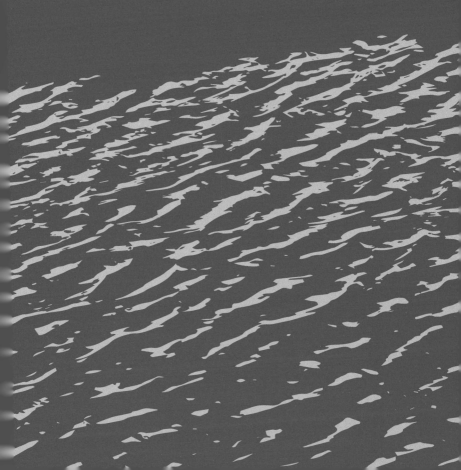

Measurement of Peritoneal Transport

Assessment of the transport function of the peritoneum used as a dialysis membrane has mainly focused on small-solute clearance, although fluid transport is more important. A standardized test for functional peritoneal assessment, the peritoneal equilibration test (PET), has been published in 1987 and widely promoted ever since. The PET consists of a 4-h dialysis exchange with a 2.27% glucose-based dialysis solution and a blood sample. Calculated parameters after drainage include the dialysate/plasma concentration ratio (D/P) of creatinine, the ratio of the dialysate glucose concentration before inflow (D_0) and after drainage (D_t/D_0), and net ultrafiltration (UF), being the difference between the drained and the instilled volume. D/P creatinine is dependent on the number of peritoneal microvessels perfused. Therefore, it represents the effective peritoneal surface area. UF failure is an important but not the only factor that can lead to overhydration. Mismatches between fluid intake, urine production, and peritoneal fluid removal are common causes for overhydration. The 2.27% glucose concentration may not be ideal for the assessment of UF capacity, because it induces only a limited quantity of ultrafiltrate. Consequently, the arousal (incomplete drainage) may overwhelm the signal (ultrafiltered volume). The 3 × 4 rule is considered the best parameter for the presence of UF failure. According to this rule, UF failure is present when net UF is <400 mL after a 4-h dwell with a 3.86%/4.25% glucose dialysis solution. Longitudinal data from the Netherlands showed that UF failure, as defined by the 3 × 4 definition, developed in <4% of patients within 2 years after the start of PD, but in 21% at some time after >2 years.

Quantification of free water transport

One hour PET, 3.86%/4.25% glucose

Na$^+$ removal = (drained volume × D$_{Na^+}$) - (instilled volume × D$_{Na^+}$)

UF small pores: Na$^+$ removal/P$_{Na^+}$ ~ Na$^+$ clearance,
which occurs through the small pores

Free water transport: total UF – UF small pores

Fig. 1. Detailed description of the calculation of free water transport. D, dialysate; P, plasma; PET, peritoneal equilibration test; UF, ultrafiltration.

Investigations into net UF assume that fluid transport occurs through a system of pores of uniform size within the vascular wall. This simplification is incorrect: UF consists of solute-coupled fluid transport through small interendothelial pores and free water transport (FWT) through endothelial aquaporin-1 (AQP-1). Glucose-induced crystalloid osmosis is required for FWT. UF during the 1st h of a dwell usually consists of 40% FWT and 60% small-pore fluid transport (Fig. 1).

A simple calculation of FWT in patients is possible with the use of a 1-h 3.86% glucose exchange. Fluid transport together with Na$^+$ transport is calculated as Na$^+$ clearance. This represents small-pore fluid transport. Subtraction of this from net UF equals FWT. However, D/P and D$_t$/D$_0$ ratios cannot be interpreted. This problem is solved with the modified (3.86% instead of 2.27% glucose) PET (MoPET) with temporary drainage after 1 h for weighing and sampling, followed by reinfusion, and final drainage after 4 h (MoPET 1/4).

It follows from the above discussion that the MoPET 1/4 is currently the best method for measurement of peritoneal transport.

Suggested Reading

Cnossen TT, Smit W, Konings CJAM, Kooman JP, Leunissen KM, Krediet RT:
Quantification of free water transport during the peritoneal equilibration test.
Perit Dial Int 2009;29:523–527.

La Milia V, Limardo M, Virga G, Crepaldi M, Locatelli F:
Simultaneous measurement of peritoneal glucose and free water
osmotic conductances.
Kidney Int 2007;72:643–650.

Parikova A, Smit W, Struijk DG, Zweers MM, Krediet RT:
The contribution of free water transport and small pore transport to the
total fluid removal in peritoneal dialysis.
Kidney Int 2005;68:1849–1856.

Sampimon DE, Coester AM, Struijk DG, Krediet RT:
The time course of peritoneal transport parameters in peritoneal dialysis
patients who develop encapsulating peritoneal sclerosis.
Nephrol Dial Transplant 2011;26:291–298.

Smit W, Struijk DG, Ho-dac-Pannekeet MM, Krediet RT:
Quantification of free water transport in peritoneal dialysis.
Kidney Int 2004;66:849–854.

Twardowski ZJ, Nolph KD, Khanna R, et al:
Peritoneal equilibration test.
Perit Dial Bull 1987;7:138–147.

Chapter 4

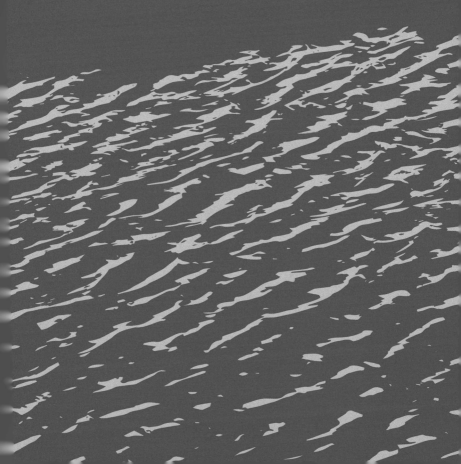

Assessment of the Peritoneum by Biomarkers in Peritoneal Effluent

Assessment of the Peritoneum by Biomarkers in Peritoneal Effluent

The effluent of peritoneal dialysis (PD) patients contains not only solutes diffused from the circulation, but also peptides and proteins that are produced by and released from peritoneal tissues. Measurement of some of these biomarkers may contribute to our insight into the status of peritoneal tissues. This is important, because serial peritoneal biopsies are impossible in patients, while nothing is known of their reproducibility. Also, morphological changes are not always reflected in parameters of peritoneal transport. The availability of ELISAs for the measurement of proteins and peptides, which can be present at low concentrations in various body fluids, created the possibility of their determination in peritoneal effluent. This created an abundancy of results without the possibility for proper interpretation. Results of proteomics contributed to the confusion, because established biomarkers were often not detected, and the functionality of some detected proteins and peptides that showed a relationship with PD duration are unknown.

Before a solute can be considered a biomarker in PD, a number of issues should be clarified, like a hypothesis on why it could reflect the status of a tissue and a confirmation of local production or release. The latter can be done by the construction of the linear relationship that is present between clearance of serum proteins that are transported from the circulation to the dialysate and their molecular weights (MW) present when plotted on a double logarithmic scale (see Chapter 1 Anatomy and Physiology of the Peritoneum). Interpolation of the clearance of a potential biomarker and its MW allows the assessment of local production on top of peritoneal transport (Fig. 1).

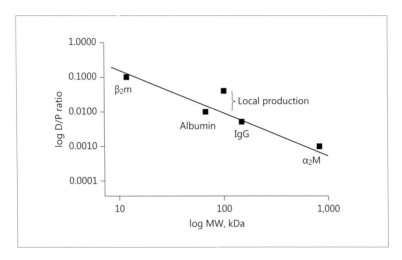

Fig. 1. Analysis of the presence of local peritoneal production/release of an effluent protein. A "transport line" is constructed on a double logarithmic scale between dialysate/plasma (D/P) ratios of selected plasma proteins and their molecular weights (MW) in every individual patient. The effluent concentrations of these proteins are likely to be determined by peritoneal transport only. The following proteins are used: β_2-microglobulin (β_2m), albumin, immunoglobulin G (IgG), and α_2-macroglobulin (α_2m). By interpolation of the potential biomarker and its MW, the presence or absence of local production/release can be assessed.

Other important issues include standardization of the dwell time and expression of the results as appearance rates (effluent concentration × volume/dwell time), because concentrations usually increase with longer dwell time. Four hours is reasonable, as a direct comparison with transport parameters is possible. Furthermore, patients should be free of peritonitis for at least 2 weeks. In general, a good biomarker should have a large intra- and a low interindividual variability. A high sensitivity and specificity should be present for the clinical outcome of interest, e.g., encapsulating peritoneal sclerosis (EPS).

Potential biomarkers can be divided into those that represent mesothelial cell mass (cancer antigen [CA]-125), cytokines (interleukin [IL]-6), growth factors (vascular endothelial growth factor [VEGF] and connective tissue growth factor (CTGF), and those that may represent tissue remodeling and peritoneal fibrosis (hyaluronan, some metalloproteinases and their inhibitors, and plasminogen activator inhibitor [PAI]-1). Some of these are irrelevant or doubtful, because the soluble form is inactive (transforming growth factor [TGF]-β), local production has not been established (CCL-18), or it is only present in the acute phase of peritonitis (tumor necrosis factor [TNF]-α).

At present, most clinical experience has been obtained with effluent CA-125, which is a large glycoprotein (MW: 220 kDa) produced by mesothelial cells. Its serum concentration is widely used as marker of ovarian carcinoma. In peritoneal tissues, it is only produced by mesothelial cells. Effluent CA-125 increases linearly with the duration of the dialysis dwell irrespective of the kind of dialysis solution. It is constitutively expressed by >70% of mesothelial cells. This is independent of PD duration. Consequently, the main use of effluent CA-125 is in the follow-up of individual patients. The intraindividual variability is 15%, which is similar to that of fluid transport parameters. The interindividual variability is 39%. A relationship between effluent CA-125 and small solute transport parameters is only present during the first 2 years of PD, probably because mesothelial cells synthesize some vasoactive substances like VEGF, especially during the mesothelial-to-mesenchymal transition. Peritonitis leads to a short, 1- to 2-fold increase in effluent CA-125. The use of "biocompatible" dialysis solutions is associated with higher CA-125 concentrations, especially when prevalent patients are switched to these. The cause is unknown, but a decrease with time on PD is present for both conventional and "biocompatible" fluids, suggesting loss of mesothelial cell mass with the duration of PD. This may explain why a low CA-125 concentration is associated with a poor PD technique survival. Patients who develop EPS have a decreased effluent CA-125 already 3 years before the clinical diagnosis, but the sensitivity and specificity for EPS are between 60 and 70%.

IL-6 is a pleiotropic cytokine with an MW of 26 kDa, which can be synthesized by various cells, e.g., mesothelial cells, macrophages, and fibroblasts. Effluent concentrations increase linearly during a dwell and exceed those in plasma, thereby proving the presence of local peritoneal production. The coefficient of intra-individual variability is 28%, but between patients it is 141%. The large day-to-day variation within an individual patient may explain the dissimilar results of analyses on relationships with peritoneal solute transport rates. This also holds through for the presence or absence of a time trend. The rise during the acute phase of peritonitis is >800 fold. The sensitivity for predicting EPS is 80%, but the specificity only 50%.

VEGF is a glycoprotein with an MW of 34 kDa that promotes angiogenesis and vascular permeability. It is a mediator of neoangiogenesis in proliferative diabetic retinopathy. Besides some diffusion from the circulation, the soluble form of VEGF is locally produced or released during PD. In vitro studies suggest that mesothelial cells are the most important source of this local production. Effluent concentrations of peritoneal VEGF are related to small solute transport parameters. Markedly increased effluent concentrations are present during mesothelial-to-mesenchymal transition and related to those of CA-125 in this condition. A relationship with the duration of PD is absent in cross-sectional analyses, but some patients show a variable increase during longitudinal follow-up. However, effluent VEGF is not a predictor for EPS.

CTGF is a cysteine-rich peptide that is involved in angiogenesis, too, but also in the expansion of the extracellular matrix. This function may be more distal from that of TGF-α. The MW of CTGF is 36 kDa, and peritoneal effluent concentrations point to local production or release. Just as for VEGF, a relationship with peritoneal small-molecular solute transport is present. However, no correlation exists between effluent CTGF and VEGF. This suggests the presence of different receptors for both growth factors.

Hyaluronan is a negatively charged unsulfated glycosaminoglycan with an MW of about 1,000 kDa. It is very hydrophilic and not bound to a core protein. Hyaluronan is an important constituent of the extracellular matrix. Results of in vitro studies have shown that cultured mesothelial cells and fibroblasts synthesize hyaluronan. The concentration of hyaluronan in peritoneal effluent is higher than that in plasma, which proves local peritoneal production. Acute peritonitis causes a >13-fold increase in effluent hyaluronan, followed by an almost immediate decrease within the first 2 days of treatment. Neither a relationship with solute transport nor a time trend is present. It is also not a predictor of EPS. The transfer of patients from conventional dialysis solutions to a "biocompatible" one is associated with a decrease in the effluent hyaluronan.

Metalloproteinase (MMP)-2 is a locally produced gelatinase with an MW of 72 kDa, which is involved in the breakdown of glycoproteins. These enzymes cleave collagens IV and V and elastin inside the basement membrane, by which they complement other collagenases in the degradation of fibrillary collagens. High effluent concentrations have been described in PD patients with alterations in peritoneal tissues, especially acute peritonitis. A cross-sectional analysis showed that the dialysate appearance rate of MMP-2 is related to small solute transport, but not to ultrafiltration, and only to a limited extent to free water transport. Some correlation with IL-6 and PAI-1 is present. No time trend is present during longitudinal follow-up. MMP-2 is also not a predictor for EPS.

PAI-1 is a glycoprotein with an MW of 50 kDa, which functions as an inhibitor of fibrinolysis. Impaired fibrinolysis is present after abdominal trauma, such as a laparotomy, and during experimental surgical peritonitis. Furthermore, elevated levels of PAI-1 are present in intra-abdominal adhesions. Besides being an inhibitor of fibrinolysis, PAI-1 is also involved in the inhibition of extracellular matrix turnover and stimulation of fibrosis, because it is upregulated by TGF-β, which is an important mediator in many fibrotic processes, like diabetic nephropathy. The peritoneal effluent PAI-1 indicates local production or release. The concentration of PAI-1 doubles transiently during acute peritonitis. A cross-sectional analysis showed relationships between effluent PAI-1 and small solute transport, ultrafiltration, and free water transport. Correlations are also present with IL-6 and MMP-2. PAI-1 is higher with longer duration of PD, which has been confirmed in a longitudinal analysis. In contrast to all other biomarkers discussed, the PAI-1 appearance rate in effluent is a powerful predictor for EPS, with a predictive power of 0.77, sensitivity of 100%, and specificity of 54%. In combination with impaired free water transport, the specificity increases to 94%.

It can be concluded that most experience has been obtained with CA-125 as a marker of mesothelial cell mass or turnover. It is especially valuable in the follow-up of individual patients. IL-6 is a good marker for peritoneal inflammation, but it is probably too sensitive, and, therefore, the results are very variable. VEGF is a marker of peritoneal angiogenesis and especially increased during endothelial-to-mesenchymal transformation of mesothelial cells. It is not a marker for imminent EPS. PAI-1 is a very promising marker for

EPS, also because it is upregulated by TGF-β and has a role in adhesion formation. However, the experience with this marker is limited, a reason to advocate further clinical studies on its use.

Suggested Reading

Krediet RT:
Dialysate cancer antigen 125 concentration as marker of peritoneal membrane status in patients treated with chronic peritoneal dialysis.
Perit Dial Int 2001;21:560–567.

Lopes Barreto D, Coester AM, Struijk DG, Krediet RT:
Can effluent matrixproteinase-2 and plasminogen activator inhibitor-1 be used as biomarkers of peritoneal membrane alterations in peritoneal dialysis patients?
Perit Dial Int 2013;33:529–537.

Lopes Barreto D, Krediet RT:
Current status and practical use of effluent biomarkers in peritoneal dialysis patients.
Am J Kidney Dis 2013;62:823–833.

Lopes Barreto D, Struijk DG, Krediet RT:
The early diagnostic potential of effluent MMP-1 and PAI-1 in encapsulating peritoneal sclerosis.
Am J Kidney Dis 2015;65:748–753.

Zweers MM, De Waart DR, Smit W, Struijk DG, Krediet RT:
The growth factors VEGF and TGF-β1 in peritoneal dialysis.
J Lab Clin Med 1999;134:124–132.

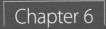
Chapter 6

Peritonitis and Other Catheter-Related Infections

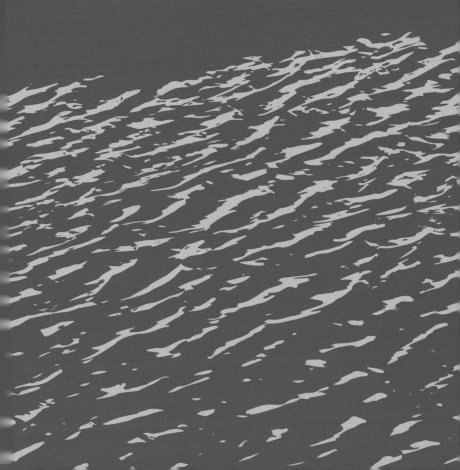

Peritonitis and Other Catheter-Related Infections

Infectious complications of peritoneal dialysis (PD) include those of the catheter exit site, the subcutaneous tunnel, and the peritoneal tissues.

Exit Site and Tunnel Infections

The presence of an exit site infection is characterized by purulent drainage with or without edema of the skin that surrounds the catheter exit. A positive culture from the exit site without the above symptoms indicates exit site colonization but not an infection. When an exit site infection extends into the subcutaneous tunnel, a tunnel infection is present. Sometimes its diagnosis is simple, for instance when the tunnel trajectory is painful, but the symptoms may also be mild. In case of doubt, an ultrasound can be helpful. *Staphylococcus aureus* and *Pseudomonas aeruginosa* are the most important causative microorganisms for the above catheter infections. Associations are present between exit site infections and subsequent peritonitis but not necessarily with the same microorganism. Treatment of catheter infections can usually be done with orally administered antibiotics, the kind of which is dependent on the causative microorganism and its sensitivity. A first-generation cephalosporin or flucloxacillin will often be the first choice. *P. aeruginosa* infections usually require treatment with 2 antibiotics for a prolonged time. A severe tunnel infection can sometimes lead to catheter removal. Patients with a double-cuffed catheter and recurrent catheter infections may benefit from shaving of the external cuff to remove the source of colonization. The incidence of exit site infections has markedly been reduced by antibiotic prophylaxis at the exit site. Both mupirocin nasal cream and gentamicin cream are used for this purpose.

Peritonitis

Definition and Diagnosis

Cloudy fluid and abdominal pain are the usual symptoms of peritonitis, but the presentation can vary widely. Fever, nausea, vomiting, weight gain due to ultrafiltration failure, diarrhea, or constipation can also be included in the presenting symptoms. Furthermore, dialysate leukocytosis can be absent or delayed, which may be due to a delayed cytokine response to infection. Therefore, awareness of the possibility of peritonitis is required in all PD patients presenting with one of these symptoms. The degree of severity is dependent on the causative organism and the etiology of peritonitis. Episodes caused by skin organisms, such as coagulase-negative staphylococci, are generally milder than peritonitis caused by *S. aureus*, streptococci, gram-negative bacteria, or fungi. Fecal peritonitis due to bowel perforation often presents with severe symptoms.

Commonly used criteria for the diagnosis of peritonitis are (1) cloudy fluid; (2) dialysate with blood cell count >100/µL; (3) polymorphonuclear cells >50%; and (4) a positive culture. Under normal conditions, the peritoneum contains not many polymorphonuclear cells. Consequently, a percentage of >50% is indicative of peritonitis, even if the absolute white cell count does not reach 100 cells/µL. To lower the incidence of culture-negative peritonitis, the number of bacteria examined in the culture should be high. Therefore, the dialysate should be centrifuged, and, to further increase test sensitivity, it should be cultured using blood culture media. Besides cultures, a Gram stain of the dialysate should be performed. Gram staining is especially useful in the diagnosis of gram-negative organisms. Overall, it is positive in 30–50% of cases. The sensitivity and specificity are lower for gram-positive organisms. However, the Gram stain may indicate the presence of yeast. Because fungal cultures might take longer to become positive, the Gram stain can allow prompt initiation of antifungal therapy.

Pathogens and Routes of Entry

Table 1 shows an overview of causes of peritonitis. PD peritonitis is commonly caused by a single positive organism. Most often this is due to contamination with gram-positive skin flora during the exchange, so-called "touch contamination." *Staphylococcus epidermidis* and *S. aureus* are cultured in the majority of these cases. Because PD patients have to perform several exchanges a day, it is not surprising that in most series gram-positive peritonitis accounts for around 50% of the peritonitis episodes.

Gram-negative peritonitis can develop due to touch contamination, exit site infection, or translocation from the bowel as a result of constipation, diverticulitis, or colitis. Gram-negative bacteria account for 20–30% of all PD-related peritonitis episodes. Peritonitis with >1 gram-negative organism and/or anaerobic peritonitis suggests bowel perforation. Polymicrobial peritonitis with gram-positive organisms can be the consequence of touch contamination or catheter infection.

Fungi are the cause of PD peritonitis in 1–13% of the episodes, and they carry a high morbidity and mortality. Most fungal infections are due to *Candida* species, especially *Candida albicans* and *C. parapsilosis*. The reasons for contamination of the dialysate with fungi are touch contamination, catheter infections, migration of

Table 1. Causes of peritonitis

Contamination
At the time of the exchange Accidental disconnection Damage to the peritoneal dialysis catheter Bites to the tubing by domestic animals
Catheter-related causes
Biofilm Exit site or tunnel infection
Enteric peritonitis
Diverticulitis Cholecystitis Bowel ischemia Colitis Gastrointestinal perforation Colonoscopy Obstipation with transmural migration of microorganisms
Hematogenous peritonitis
After dental procedures Infected foreign body
Gynecological causes
After gynecological procedures Vaginal leak of dialysate Use of intrauterine devices Vaginal labor

fungi across the bowel wall into the peritoneum, intestinal perforation, and fistulae from the vagina to the peritoneum.

Mycobacterium peritonitis is rare. The clinical presentation is indistinguishable from nontuberculous bacterial peritonitis. Awareness is especially required when the patient is living in an endemic area and has a culture-negative refractory peritonitis.

Differential Diagnosis of a Cloudy Effluent

Most often cloudy effluent is due to infectious peritonitis. However, there are other possible causes, e.g., when the dialysate sample is taken from a dry abdomen. Another etiology of cloudy effluent is chemical peritonitis, also called sterile peritonitis, which may be the result of drug toxicity (vancomycin and amphotericin, some dihydropyridine calcium channel blockers), or a reaction to icodextrin dialysis solution in earlier days. In this case, stopping the drug or icodextrin will clear the dialysate. Chylous ascites due to triglyceride or lipid leakage is a rare cause of cloudy effluent. It can be related to lymphatic obstruction due to malignancy (especially lymphoma) or acute pancreatitis. Eosinophilia of the effluent (>10% eosinophils) can be present due to an allergic reaction in response to the plastic dialysate bags or the plasticizers in the PD catheter. Icodextrin has also been associated with increased eosinophils in the dialysate. In most cases, the eosinophils disappear without treatment. Blood-stained effluent can be caused by trauma of the abdomen, ovulation, due to a ruptured ectopic pregnancy, uterine rupture, or vascular accidents, such as rupture of an aneurysm.

Differential Diagnosis of Culture-Negative Peritonitis

Culture technique problems are an important cause of culture-negative peritonitis. In addition, recent use of antibiotics may result in some antibiotic activity in the dialysate, with negative cultures as a consequence. Another explanation for negative cultures is difficult-to-culture organisms, such as mycobacteria or fungi. The microbiologist should be aware of this and use special culture methods to identify these organisms. Due to better and improved culture techniques, the incidence of culture-negative peritonitis has decreased in time. The International Society for Peritoneal Dialysis (ISPD) states that the incidence of culture-negative peritonitis may not exceed 15%. Higher rates suggest problems with the culture techniques used.

Terminology

Four different entities of peritonitis can be distinguished. Recurrent peritonitis is an episode of peritonitis that occurs within 4 weeks of completion of therapy of a prior episode but with a different organism. In relapsing peritonitis, an episode of peritonitis with the same organism occurs within 4 weeks after completion of therapy of a prior episode. This is mostly due to a subcutaneous tunnel infection, a catheter biofilm in the lumen of the PD catheter, or inadequate treatment of the prior peritonitis. When the effluent is cleared of white cells, it is possible to replace the PD catheter instead of removing it. In this way, a temporary switch to hemodialysis can be avoided. Repeated peritonitis is an episode that occurs 4 weeks after therapy completion of a prior episode with the same organism. Finally, refractory peritonitis is defined as failure of the effluent to become clear after 5 days of antibiotic therapy. In this situation, catheter removal is always indicated. Delayed removal of the PD catheter leads to increased mortality and has a high risk of peritoneal membrane failure when the patient returns to PD.

Treatment

When peritonitis is suspected, and Gram stain and cultures are taken, antibiotic therapy should be started promptly. Delay in therapy may have severe consequences, i.e., relapsing peritonitis, catheter removal, technique failure, or death. Empiric antibiotics must cover both gram-positive and -negative organisms. For gram-positive coverage, either a first-generation cephalosporin or vancomycin can be used, and for gram-negative coverage either a third-generation cephalosporin or an aminoglycoside will prove suitable. The ISPD recommends center-specific selection of empiric therapy, dependent on the local history of organisms and their sensitivities. The preferred route of antibiotic administration is intraperitoneal, because this brings the drug directly to the site of action. Moreover, it allows a patient who does not need hospitalization to be treated at home. Intravenous or oral administration is only possible for antibiotics with a low protein binding, because only the free fraction is transported from the systemic circulation to the dialysis fluid. When culture results are known, the antibiotic treatment can be adjusted to narrow-spectrum agents according to the resistance of the causative organism. Culture-negative peritonitis is mostly due to gram-positive organisms. Therefore, it is reasonable to stop gram-negative-directed therapy on day 3 of treatment when the patient is doing well. Only gram-positive coverage should then be continued for 14 days.

Dose adjustment for residual renal function is not necessary. When the patient is known to have a fast peritoneal transport rate, with a higher clearance from the dialysate, it may be better to use higher antibiotic dosing. Both intermittent (once a day, with a minimal dwell duration of 6 h) or continuous dosing (in each dwell) can be used.

Most patients with PD-related peritonitis will show clinical improvement within 48 h after the initiation of treatment. When clinical improvement is absent, cell counts and cultures should be repeated. In addition, reevaluation for the existence of an exit site or tunnel infection, or intra-abdominal abscess should be done. If peritonitis co-insides with an exit site or tunnel infection, catheter removal should be considered. In general, catheter removal is advised when there is no clinical improvement after 5 days of appropriate antibiotic therapy.

The duration of the antibiotic therapy depends on the causative organism. In case of *S. epidermidis* and culture-negative peritonitis, 14 days of therapy will be sufficient. With *S. aureus, Enterococcus,* and gram-negative organisms, 21-day treatment is advised. The ISPD states that ideally repeated cell counts and cultures of the effluent should guide the duration of therapy. Table 2 shows an overview of the specific organisms with their most common etiology, presentation, outcome, and treatment duration.

Incidence and Prevention

An ISPD guideline states that a center's peritonitis rate should be no more than 1 episode every 18 months. In the early days of PD, patients had peritonitis, on average, every 10 weeks. The use of a Y-set disconnect system and the "flush-before-fill" technique in the 1980s led to a dramatic decrease in the peritonitis rate. Even 1 episode in every 33 patient-months has been reported. With this technique, some fresh dialysate is washed out into the drainage bag, flushing out any bacteria that might have contaminated the tubing at the time of the connection. The next step is drainage of the dialysate into the empty bag, followed by filling of the abdominal cavity with the new solution.

In an attempt to further reduce the incidence of PD-related infections, the use of prophylactic measures has been implemented in clinical patient care. The use of prophylactic antibiotics at the time of insertion of the PD catheter is one of these measures. A single dose of intravenous antibiotic administered before catheter placement decreases the risk of a subsequent infection. A first-generation cephalosporin has been most frequently used for this purpose. A single dose of vancomycin may be more effective, but it must be

Table 2. Survey of peritonitis

Organism	Etiology	Presentation	Outcome	Treatment duration
Coagulase-negative staphylococci	Touch contamination	Mild clinical symptoms	Respond well to treatment Relapsing peritonitis due to biofilm: catheter replacement during antibiotic therapy	2 weeks
Enterococcus species	Intra-abdominal pathology	Severe peritonitis	>1 organism in 50%: associated with catheter removal, permanent transfer to HD, death	3 weeks
Streptococcus	Dental source *S. bovis*: colon	Severe peritonitis	Respond well to treatment	2 weeks
Staphylococcus aureus	Touch contamination, catheter problems	Severe peritonitis	Associated with catheter or colonization; often requires catheter removal	3 weeks
Coryne-bacterium	Touch contamination	Mild clinical symptoms	Respond well to treatment	3 weeks
Culture-negative peritonitis	Preceded by treatment Often gram-positive bacteria	Mild clinical symptoms	Day 3: improvement, stop gram-negative but continue gram-positive coverage No response: use special culture techniques No response on day 5: catheter removal	3 weeks
Pseudomonas	Often associated with catheter infection	Severe peritonitis	Associated with more hospitalization, catheter removal, transfer to HD Association with catheter infection	3 weeks
Steno-trophomonas	Often preceded by antibiotic treatment	Less severe than *Pseudomonas*	Often not associated with catheter infection	3 weeks

Table 2 (continued)

Organism	Etiology	Presentation	Outcome	Treatment duration
Other single gram-negative organisms	Touch contamination Exit site infection Translocation (constipation, diverticulitis, colitis)	Severe peritonitis	Higher death rate, hospitalization, catheter loss, transfer to HD than gram-positive peritonitis Treatment failure: catheter biofilm: catheter removal	2 weeks
>1 gram-negative organism	Intra-abdominal pathology (especially in combination with anaerobic bacteria)	Severe peritonitis	Surgical evaluation High mortality	3 weeks
>1 gram-positive organism	Touch contamination Catheter problems	Mild	Respond well to treatment	3 weeks
Fungal peritonitis	Often preceded by antibiotics	Severe peritonitis	High hospitalization rates, catheter loss, transfer to HD, death Catheter removal!	2–4 weeks
Myco-bacterium	Endemic area Immuno-suppressed patients	Mild-severe peritonitis	Difficult diagnosis: consider in patients with refractory or relapsing peritonitis with negative cultures Catheter removal not always necessary	12–18 months
HD, hemodialysis.				

administered slowly to reduce the risk of ototoxicity and to avoid an infusion reaction (known as the "red man syndrome").

Several studies have shown that *S. aureus* nasal carriage increases the risk of peritonitis as well as exit site and tunnel infections. A systemic review on topical mupirocin treatment, intranasally or at the exit site, concluded its effectiveness in preventing exit site infection and peritonitis. A comparison between mupirocin and gentamicin at the exit site showed similar results for S. *aureus*, but gentamicin was more effective prophylaxis for gram-negative organisms. However, it is quite possible that more resistance will occur in the long run.

A Cochrane systematic review has shown that the type of catheter used, i.e., a Tenckhoff catheter or a swan neck catheter, does not influence the peritonitis rate. The same holds true for a comparison between continuous ambulatory and automated PD. Hence, the choice for one of these therapy options should not be based on a difference in peritonitis risk.

Prophylactic antibiotics can be considered to prevent peritonitis after several procedures: e.g., colonoscopy, hysteroscopy, and dental procedures, after connection problems. However, good evidence and the optimal antibiotic regimen is missing. Peritonitis with fungi and yeasts is usually preceded by prior antibiotic use.

Highly inconsistent data have been reported about the use of biocompatible solutions compared to conventional solutions and their effect on peritonitis incidence. Recently, a systematic review has been performed about this issue. It showed that the use of biocompatible solutions did not result in a decline in peritonitis episodes.

Outcome

Most peritonitis episodes resolve with antibiotics; percentages from 60 to 90% are reported in the literature. The cure rate is higher when there is no simultaneous tunnel or exit site infection. The causative organism is also of importance. In comparison with

Table 3. Indications for catheter removal

Established	To be considered
Refractory peritonitis	Repeat peritonitis
Relapsing peritonitis	Mycobacterial peritonitis
Fungal peritonitis	Peritonitis with >1 gram-negative organism
Refractory exit site and tunnel infection	

gram-positive organisms, catheter removal rates are higher with peritonitis caused by gram-negative organisms or fungi. Abdominal wall or intra-abdominal abscess formation is a rare complication of peritonitis (<1%). Drainage of the abscess is indicated. Peritonitis is a major cause of temporary or permanent transfer to hemodialysis (technique failure). In a Dutch multicenter study, peritonitis accounted for 10–18% of technique failure during the first 3 years of PD. Death occurs in 1–6% of episodes. The mortality is higher for peritonitis due to gram-negative organisms (4–10%) and fungi (20–45%).

Indications for Catheter Removal

The indications for catheter removal are listed in Table 3. Preservation of the peritoneal membrane is always more important than salvation of the PD catheter. In cases of relapsing peritonitis, the infected catheter should be removed, but it can be replaced as a simultaneous procedure when the effluent leukocyte count is low during adequate antibiotic therapy. If the peritonitis does not respond within 5 days of adequate antibiotic therapy, the catheter should be removed immediately. Simultaneous insertion of a new catheter is prohibited under these circumstances. The same applies to fungal peritonitis. The optimal time period between catheter removal and insertion is not known. In the literature, 2–3 weeks is recommended, even longer in the case of fungal peritonitis.

Suggested Reading

Li PK, Szeto CC, Piraino B, de Arteaga J, Fan S, Figueiredo AE, Fish DN,
Goffin E, Kim YL, Salzer W, Struijk DG, Teitelbaum I, Johnson DW:
ISPD peritonitis recommendations: 2016 update on prevention and treatment.
Perit Dial Int 2016;36:481–508.

Szeto CC, Li PK, Johnson DW, Bernardini J, Dong J, Figueiredo AE,
Ito Y, Kazancioglu R, Moraes T, Van Esch S, Brown EA:
ISPD catheter-related infection recommendations: 2017 update.
Perit Dial Int 2017;37:141–154.

Van Esch S, Krediet RT, Struijk DG:
32-years of experience in peritoneal dialysis-related peritonitis
in a university hospital.
Perit Dial Int 2014;34:162–170.

Chapter 7

Information Technology in Peritoneal Dialysis

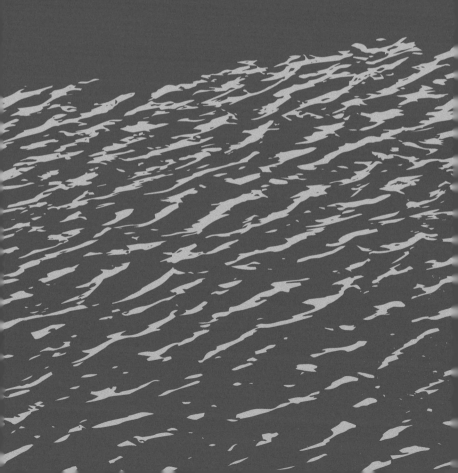

Information Technology in Peritoneal Dialysis

Peritoneal dialysis (PD) is a home-based dialysis mode. This implies that the treatment itself is ideally performed by the patient. However, when the patient is (no longer) able to take care of their dialysis, their partner, other relatives, friends, or district nurses have to support the treatment. Although the treatment is not extremely complex, questions may arise that need to be answered. Nowadays, this is still usually done either by calling the dialysis department or by visiting an outpatient clinic. Especially in rural areas, the latter can result in long travel distances. To improve patient support as well as patient care, information technology (IT) can be used for improving patient contact using video conversation and all kinds of devices for remote monitoring. In this chapter, a summary is given on the potential benefits of applying IT to PD patients as well as an overview of the studies on IT in this population.

Potential Benefits

For the patient, IT can help in improving self-management, support the treatment at home, and give a feeling of safety. It might help in reducing outpatient clinic visits or even prevent hospitalization. For the health care provider, IT can improve patient care, can increase the number of frail patients treated at home, and, at the same time, save time and money by reducing outpatient clinic visits and hospitalization.

Telemedicine

Telemedicine is the use of IT to provide clinical health care at a distance. It helps eliminate distance barriers and can improve access to medical services that would often not be consistently available in distant rural communities. PD patients who live far away from their medical facility are indeed at risk. In a study in Canada, technique failure and death rate were investigated in relation to the distance the patients lived from the nephrologist. They showed that the risk of technique failure increased with increasing distance to the closest nephrologist. Also, in PD patients living 50 to >300 km from the closest nephrologist, the risk of death was significantly increased compared to those living within 50 km of their nephrologist. Adjustment for physician supply nearby did not influence our results, suggesting that reduced access to local primary care physicians or non-nephrologist specialists was not responsible for the increased risk of death among remote residents.

Videoconferencing

The use of videoconferencing has been evaluated in the long-term control of stable patients undergoing PD at home. In a randomized setup, 25 patients using videoconferencing were compared to 32 control patients during a mean of 8 months. The study patients were followed using alternate months of teleconsultations and hospital visits. On average, 22 min were spent on each teleconsultation, which was significantly less than in hospital consultations, which lasted on average 33 min. In 148 out of a total of 172 teleconsultations (89%), medical treatment was modified. In only 4 cases (2%), patients needed an additional hospital visit. In all teleconsultations, the condition of the catheter exit site and the presence of edema could be evaluated. The estimated cost of telemedicine was EUR 198 and that of a hospital visit was EUR 177. The mean hospitalization rate in the videoconferencing group was 2.2 days/patient/year, which was significantly lower than the 5.7 days in the patients without teleconsultations.

Software has been developed in India that not only enabled videoconferencing but also facilitated the recording of details about PD exchanges, taking images, and audiovisual depictions to show patients each step of a PD exchange. The authors compared 115 patients who used this software in a rural area to 131 urban patients during a follow-up of about 1.5 years. Both groups showed similar technique survival, peritonitis rates, and exit site infections. The rural patients had a better survival (43 vs. 30 months, $p < 0.05$). In another study, they compared the quality of life and socioeconomic-related parameters. No differences in quality of life were revealed. However, rural patients had a significantly reduced number of visits to the hospital, fewer hospitalized days, and fewer nephrologist consultations.

Telemonitoring (Real Time)
Real-time monitoring of patient vital signs and direct provision of care in continuous ambulatory PD patients was employed using a cellular telephone and an internet web site by Nakamoto [2007]. All data for the patients – blood pressure, heart rate, body weight, ultrafiltration volume, and urine volume – were collected in real time and sent directly to the treating physician's office over the Internet. Abnormal data are shown in the host computer with an emergency signal (emergency alarm system). This system also facilitated contact to the medical staff. Lew et al. [2017] monitored blood pressure and weight in 269 PD patients. They concluded that remote biometric monitoring was feasible and increased communication between patients and providers. Another study looked at patient satisfaction during a 15-month study using a tablet to record vital data (weight,

blood pressure, dialysis exchanges, and ultrafiltration volume) combining a set of questions on PD-related complaints. Satisfaction scores and retention rates suggested a high level of acceptability.

A PD-specific tool is the remote monitoring of the PD cycler. This was already available in the beginning of this century by connecting the cycler using a modem to software in the dialysis unit (PD Link; Baxter Healthcare Corporation, Deerfield, IL, USA). It was also possible to transport the data to the dialysis unit using a memory card. Recently, a remote patient management tool has been introduced that uses cloud-based connectivity and enables remote monitoring as well as remote programming of the cycler (Claria-Sharesource; Baxter Healthcare Corporation). Although this tool might help in improving patient satisfaction and patient outcomes and saving costs, this needs to be confirmed in further studies. Until now, only a simulation study was performed by 11 automated PD teams in 12 automated PD patient profiles by Makhija et al. [2018]. They estimated that 2-way remote monitoring could reduce health care resource utilization.

Conclusions

In PD, still only limited data are available on the use of IT. However, the available data on videoconferencing and telemonitoring are promising. In general, conclusive evidence is still lacking. Further research is needed to confirm the cost-effectiveness of the use of IT in this patient population.

Suggested Reading

Chand DH, Bednarz D:
Daily remote peritoneal dialysis monitoring: an adjunct to enhance patient care.
Perit Dial Int 2008;28:533–537.

Dey V, Jones A, Spalding EM:
Telehealth: acceptability, clinical interventions and quality
of life in peritoneal dialysis.
SAGE Open Med 2016;10:1–6.

Drepper VJ, Martin P-Y, Chopard CS, Sload JA:
Remote patient management in automated peritoneal dialysis:
a promising new tool.
Perit Dial Int 2018;38:76–78.

Gallar P, Vigil A, Rodriguez I, Ortega O, Gutierrez M, Hurtado J, et al:
Two-year experience with telemedicine in the follow-up of
patients in home peritoneal dialysis.
J Telemed Telecare 2007;13:288–292.

Lew SQ, Sikka N, Thompson C, Cherian T, Magnus M:
Adoption of telehealth: remote biometric monitoring among
peritoneal dialysis patients in the United States.
Perit Dial Int 2017;37:576–578.

Makhija D, Alscher MD, Becker S, et al:
Remote monitoring of automated peritoneal dialysis patients: assessing clinical and
economic value.
Telemed J E Health 2018;24:1–9.

Nakamoto H:
Telemedicine system for patients on continuous ambulatory peritoneal dialysis.
Perit Dial Int 2007;27(suppl 2):S21–S26.

Nayak Karopadi A, Antony S, Subhramanayam SV, Nayak KS:
Remote monitoring of peritoneal dialysis: Why? Where? How?
Hong Kong J Nephrol 2013;15:6–13.

Tonelli M, Hemmelgarn B, Culleton B, Klarenbach S, et al:
Mortality of Canadians treated by peritoneal dialysis in remote locations.
Kidney Int 2007;72:1023–1028.

Chapter 7

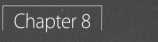

Residual Renal Function and Peritoneal Dialysis Dose in Adequacy of Peritoneal Dialysis

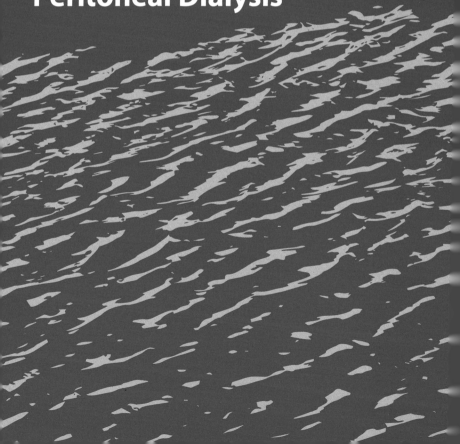

Residual Renal Function and Peritoneal Dialysis Dose in Adequacy of Peritoneal Dialysis

The development of continuous ambulatory peritoneal dialysis (CAPD) in the end-70s enabled nephrologists to observe a better preservation of residual kidney function with CAPD than to hemodialysis (HD). This observation was first published from France already in 1984 and confirmed in many other studies since, including the Netherlands Cooperative Study on the Adequacy of Dialysis (NECOSAD), which also shows that high blood pressure, comorbidity, and hypovolemia are associated with this decline. No marked differences are present between automated PD and CAPD.

The excretory kidney function consists of glomerular filtration and tubular secretion and reabsorption. In the presence of normal kidney function, about 99% of the glomerular filtrate is reabsorbed. Consequently, urine production is not influenced by the glomerular filtration rate (GFR) but by tubular transport mechanisms. A different situation is present in PD patients, in whom urine volume accounts for half of the variance in GFR. Apparently, tubuloglomerular feedback mechanisms are disturbed or function differently in dialysis patients.

Inulin clearance is the gold standard for GFR determination in humans, but its determination is cumbersome. Creatinine clearance overestimates GFR due to some tubular secretion and that of urea gives an underestimation because of reabsorption, especially in the presence of hypovolemia. The mean of urea and creatinine clearance is closely related to inulin clearance in dialysis patients. Therefore, the mean of both clearances can be considered the reference method for GFR determination in this population. However, it requires a timed and accurate urine collection.

Formulae have been developed for GFR estimation based on plasma concentrations of creatinine and urea to avoid cumbersome urine collections. The modification of diet in renal disease (MDRD) equation is widely used and extensively validated but not in (pre)dialysis patients. It consists of gender and race in the numerator and creatinine and age in the denominator. Despite the reasonable results of the MDRD formula in patients with a GFR between 20 and 60 mL/min, a number of studies, including an analysis by the ERA-EDTA (European Renal Association-European Dialysis and Transplant Association) registry, report higher mortality of patients who start dialysis with the highest estimated GFR values, despite extensive corrections for potentially confounding factors. The explanation of this unexpected finding is the dependency of plasma creatinine on muscle mass, which is more important for death than the effect of glomerular filtration in a situation of dialysis initiation.

A high plasma concentration of urea is generally considered a representation of uremic toxicity in nondialyzed patients with chronic renal failure, despite the fact that it is not toxic. Urea and creatinine are small molecules and therefore easily removed from the body by dialysis techniques, where diffusion is the main transport mechanism. The removal of unmeasured larger molecules and protein-bound toxins by dialysis is almost absent or much lower. This contrasts to native kidneys that remove solutes by glomerular filtration and tubular secretion, both not influenced by their molecular weight. It follows from this reasoning that plasma urea is a poor marker of uremic toxicity in patients treated with chronic dialysis. Yet, adequacy of dialysis is usually defined by the clearance of urea (Kt/V_{urea}), while in PD the clearance of creatinine is also used (weekly creatinine clearance/1.73 m^2 body surface area).

Targets for solute removal in PD have first been formulated in 1997 by the Dialysis Outcomes Quality Initiative (DOQI) and are intended for use in the USA. They comprise the following targets: Kt/V_{urea} 2.0/week and weekly creatinine clearance 60 L/1.73 m^2. In comparison, an average CAPD patient has a peritoneal Kt/V_{urea} of 1.5–1.7 and a peritoneal creatinine clearance of 40–45 L/week. These recommendations are based on results from the CANUSA (Canada-USA) study and have been extremely harmful for further PD development. This study included 680 new PD patients from Canada and the USA and showed that higher overall solute clearances were associated with better survival. However, the mean follow-up of only 15 months makes confounding by residual renal function a likely explanation for the superior survival. No other study reported an effect of peritoneal solute clearances on mortality. A re-analysis of the CANUSA study also showed that mortality was not associated with peritoneal clearance but only with urine production. The importance of residual renal function was confirmed in the NECOSAD cohort, not only concerning patient survival but also for patients' perceived quality of life. Therefore, a Kt/V_{urea} <1.7 in the absence of uremic complaints is not a reason to transfer a PD patient to HD. The lack of evidence for the DOQI recommendations has been established firmly in 2 randomized controlled trials from Mexico and Hong-Kong. Both were unable to detect any effect of increasing peritoneal solute clearances reaching the DOQI targets on patient survival, not even in anuric patients. So, it is clear that pushing up peritoneal Kt/V_{urea} from 1.6 to 2.0 per week in patients without signs of underdialysis has no effect on their survival: the effect of peritoneal solute clearance is overpowered by that of residual renal function.

Evidently, a minimum dialysis dose is required in anuric patients. For ethical reasons, this cannot be investigated in a randomized controlled trial. A NECOSAD analysis showed that only Kt/V_{urea} <1.5 and creatinine clearance <40 L/week are associated with increased mortality. Both targets are easily achieved with CAPD. Only few patients with a slow solute transport who are treated with an automated PD scheme consisting of many short (e.g., 30-min) exchanges can have a discrepancy between a normal Kt/V and a creatinine clearance <40 L/week. These patients often have clinical signs of underdialysis.

All discussed data show evidently that the emphasis on peritoneal solute clearances is a misconception due to neglectance of the importance of residual kidney function. Whether the most important contribution to mortality reduction of residual kidney function is the quantity of urine production which minimizes the risk of overhydration, tubular function allowing better removal of large and protein-bound solutes, or any endocrine function is currently not established. Maintenance of kidney function is probably an important reason for the superior survival of PD patients compared to those treated with HD.

Suggested Reading

Grootendorst DG, Michels WM, Richardson JD, Jager KJ, Boescoten EW,
Dekker FW, Krediet RT, et al:
The MDRD formula does not reflect GFR in ESRD patients.
Nephrol Dial Transplant 2011;26:1932–1937.

Jansen MAM, Hart AAM, Korevaar JC, Dekker FW, Boeschoten EW,
Krediet RT, et al:
Predictors of the decline rate of residual renal function in incident dialysis patients.
Kidney Int 2002;62:1046–1053.

Jansen MAM, Termorshuizen F, Korevaar JC, Dekker FW, Boeschoten EW,
Krediet RT; NECOSAD Study Group:
Predictors of survival in anuric peritoneal dialysis patients.
Kidney Int 2005;68:1199–1205.

Krediet RT, Dekker FW:
Can plasma creatinine levels guide initiation of dialysis?
Nat Rev Nephrol 2010;6:563–564.

Krediet RT:
Preservation of residual kidney function and urine volume in patients on dialysis.
Clin J Am Soc Nephrol 2017;12:377–379.

Panigua R, Amato D, Vonesh E, Correa-Rotter, Ramos A, Moran J, Mujais S:
Effects of increased peritoneal clearances on mortality rates in peritoneal
dialysis: ADEMEX, a prospective, randomized, controlled trial.
J Am Soc Nephrol 2002;13:1307–1320.

Termorshuizen F, Korevaar JC, Dekker FW, van Maanen JG, Boeschoten EW,
Krediet RT, et al:
The relative importance of residual renal function compared with peritoneal
clearance for patient survival and quality of life: an analysis of the Netherlands
Cooperative Study on the Adequacy of Dialysis (NECOSAD)-2.
Am J Kidney Dis 2003;41:1293–1302.

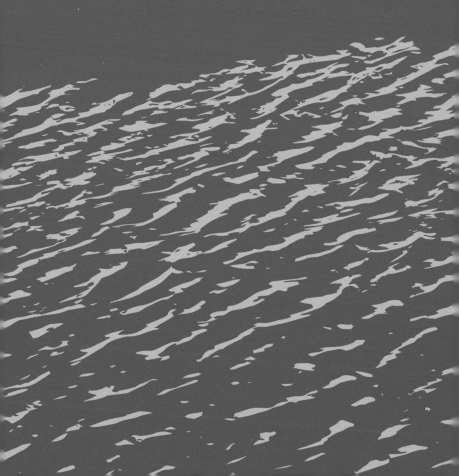

Chapter 9
Peritoneal Dialysis Solutions

Peritoneal Dialysis Solutions

The conventional fluids used for peritoneal dialysis (PD) that are commercially available consist of a lactate-buffered, positively charged electrolyte solution that contains large amounts of glucose to induce a crystalloid osmotic pressure gradient between the peritoneal cavity and the peritoneal microvasculature. These solutions, which were already available in the 70s of the last century, contain no potassium, and they have variable concentrations of calcium and magnesium. Their pH is 5.5, which is required to prevent caramelization of glucose during heat sterilization. Heat sterilization is legally required but induces the formation of advanced glycosylation end products (AGE), mainly aldehydes and dicarbonyl compounds. The solutions are delivered in plastic bags, which have a device for the addition of additives, e.g., antibiotics. The composition of a typical conventional dialysis solution is given in Table 1.

It follows from the composition that these solutions resemble the extracellular fluid to a limited extent only. The main differences are the absence of proteins, the acidity, lactate, hyperosmolality, and, most strikingly, the extremely high glucose concentrations, which are far above the range seen in diabetic patients with a hyperglycemic dysregulation. Nevertheless, the use of these conventional solutions is well tolerated by most patients. Only after prolonged use, i.e., >2 years, permanent alterations can develop in peritoneal morphology and transport. The bioincompatibility of the conventional solutions has led to the development of solutions aimed to replace glucose and solutions aimed to deal with the acidity and glucose degradation products (GDP).

Amino acid-based dialysis solutions have been developed to replace glucose. The aim was to use their absorption during a dialysis

Table 1. Composition of some commercially available dialysis solutions

Constituent	Concentration
Na$^+$, mmol/L	132
K$^+$, mmol/L	0
Ca^{2+}, mmol/L	1.25, 1.75
Mg^{2+}, mmol/L	0.25, 0.75
Cl$^-$, mmol/L	102
Lactate, mmol/L[a]	35, 40
Glucose, mmol/L[b]	75, 125, 214
Glucose, g/L[c]	13.6/15.0, 22.7/25.0, 38.6/42.5
Osmolality, mosm/kg H$_2$O	334, 397, 486

[a] Some solutions contain D-lactate, others a racemic mixture.
[b] Some solutions contain D-glucose (dextrose), others a mixture of D- and L-glucose.
[c] Differences are dependent on the use of the European or American pharmacopoeia, but the concentrations in mmol/L are not different.

exchange as an additional source of nitrogen. The loss of proteins and amino acids that occurs during PD due to diffusion from the circulation to the dialysate was the rationale. The use of amino acid-based solutions is limited to 1 exchange/day to prevent an extensive nitrogen load on the body, because the absorption of amino acids averages 70% during a 4-h dwell. The results obtained with a 1.1% solution on parameters of nutritional status are not impressive, but the solution is still used to reduce peritoneal exposure to glucose. Consequently, the osmolality is similar to that of a 1.36% glucose-based solution and thus unable to remove excess fluid from the body in most patients.

Icodextrin is the only high-molecular-weight osmotic agent that is currently available. It is a mixture of glucose polymer fractions of

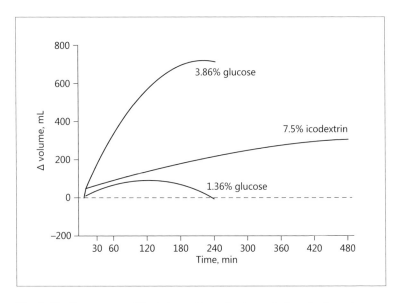

Fig. 1. The time course of the intraperitoneal volume during single exchanges of a 1.36% glucose solution, a 3.86% glucose solution, and a 7.5% icodextrin solution. Taken from *Nolph and Gokal's Textbook of Peritoneal Dialysis* [2009] and published with permission of Springer.

hydrolyzed cornstarch with a mean molecular weight of 16 kDa, which is available as a 7.5% lactate-buffered solution. The solution has an osmolality of 284 mosm/kg H_2O and induces a colloid osmotic pressure gradient, which is in contrast to the crystalloid pressure gradient brought about by low-molecular-weight osmotic agents. The pH is 5.8, and it contains a smaller amount of glucose degradation products than all glucose-based dialysis solutions. Icodextrin is especially effective during an 8- to 12-h dwell, because the peritoneal absorption rate is low (Fig. 1).

Chapter 9

Icodextrin induces especially high ultrafiltration in patients with fast transport of low-molecular-weight solutes, indicating the presence of a large effective peritoneal surface area. In this situation, many pores are available for ultrafiltration. With glucose-based solutions, this effect is counteracted by a high absorption rate of glucose, leading to a rapid disappearance of the crystalloid osmotic pressure gradient. This is not the case for icodextrin. The difference in the absorption rates of glucose and icodextrin explains why acute peritonitis leads to reduced ultrafiltration on glucose-based solutions and increased fluid removal on icodextrin. The small amount of icodextrin absorbed is degraded to maltose by circulating amylase. In the presence of a normal kidney function, maltose is removed from the body by glomerular filtration, followed by uptake and degradation in the proximal tubule. The only way to remove maltose in dialysis patients is transport to the intracellular space, where breakdown by maltase occurs. Due to the absence of removal by the kidneys, the use of icodextrin is limited to 1 long exchange per day. With this policy, plasma maltose stabilizes at around 3 mmol/L and total carbohydrate at around 0.3 mmol/L.

Reported side effects of icodextrin include skin rashes, which are infrequent, and an epidemic of culture-negative peritonitis that occurred in 2002, which was caused by contamination with peptidoglycans. These are substances present in the cell wall of bacteria that can contaminate corn and are not removed by heat sterilization. Culture-negative peritonitis disappeared after the production process had been modified reducing the peptidoglycan content to below detection limits. Icodextrin also influences some clinical chemistry investigations, like plasma Na^+, some glucose determination methods, and plasma amylase. Plasma Na^+ is on average 2–3 mmol/L lower than in patients not on icodextrin. This is a compensation for the contribution of maltose to plasma osmolality. Interference of icodextrin metabolites with some self-control glucose methods can lead to falsely increased readings of blood glucose concentrations, especially with glucose dehydrogenase methods. The use of icodextrin leads to unexplained low plasma amylase concentrations, which can be problematic when pancreatitis is suspected.

Biocompatibility can be defined as the ability of material, object, or system to function without an important host reaction in a specific situation. The conventional PD solutions are bioincompatible, because they influence peritoneal morphology and transport, especially after prolonged exposure. The morphological alterations that can develop in long-term PD patients consist of neoangiogenesis with diabetiform vascular changes and subendothelial hyalinosis, loss of mesothelial cells, and fibrotic alterations, both submesothelially and in the interstitium in general. Extensive deposition of collagen is a late event that can develop after several years of PD. In contrast, peritoneal AGE deposition occurs already after some months of PD treatment, which is also the case for mesothelial-to-mesenchymal transition.

Conventional dialysis solutions have a number of factors that can explain their bioincompatibility, like their acidity, hyperosmolality, the buffer, extremely high glucose concentrations, and GDP presence, but their relative importance in the pathogenesis of peritoneal alterations in PD patients has not been established. Attempts to increase biocompatibility of dialysis solutions have focused mainly on increasing the pH, the buffer substance, and decreasing GDP concentrations. Cell cultures have mostly been the major outcome parameter, meaning that results in these models are not always important in the clinical situation. This can be illustrated by the harmful effects of exposure of an acid dialysis solution to cell cultures, because it lowers the intracellular pH. Patients always have a residual dialysate volume after drainage of 200–300 mL. This has a nor-

Table 2. Currently available biocompatible peritoneal dialysis solutions

Name	pH	Buffer	3-DG, μmol/L	Producer
Physioneal	7.4	Bicarbonate lactate	253	Baxter
Balance	7.0	Lactate	–	Fresenius
Bicavera	7.4	Bicarbonate	42	Fresenius
3-DG, 3-deoxyglucosone, a glucose degradation product.				

mal pH and leads to immediate dilution of the instilled fresh dialysis fluid, which raises the pH to 7 within 10–15 min.

Preparation of biocompatible dialysis solutions requires a double-bag system, in which one bag contains the electrolytes and glucose at a very low pH and the other one the buffer. Heat sterilization at a low pH reduces GDP formation. GDP promote AGE formation at a faster speed than glucose in in vitro studies. Both bags are mixed before inflow into the patient. Table 2 summarizes the differences between the currently available biocompatible dialysis solutions.

Studies in cell cultures have shown improvements in cell viability compared to exposure to conventional dialysis solutions, and ex vivo macrophages in peritoneal effluent have better preservation of their functions. Long-term exposure of rats to Physioneal® reduces the amount of peritoneal fibrosis to some extent compared to conventional solutions. A similar effect was also observed in a study in patients. Clinical studies all show reduced inflow pain and higher effluent concentrations of cancer antigen 125 (CA-125), suggesting a favorable effect on the mesothelium. No effects are present on peritoneal transport. Only one study comparing Balance® with Stay Safe® (a conventional solution) reported the absence of the slight rise in the dialysate/plasma ratio of creatinine in Balance® that occurred in Stay Safe® after 2 years. No effects were found on ultrafiltration in this study. Some investigations reported a slight decrease in serum concentrations of circulating AGE, but the relevance of this finding is unknown. Results of studies on the occurrence of peritonitis are equivocal. Good investigations into the time course of residual renal function have shown no effect. Despite lower mortality rates on biocompatible solutions in uncontrolled studies reported, this phenomenon could not be confirmed in a randomized controlled trial.

It can be concluded that the main advantage of amino acid-based solutions is their ability to reduce peritoneal exposure to glucose and GDPs, while their effect on nutritional status is minimal. Icodextrin also reduces glucose exposure, and it is the only dialysis solution with a high-molecular-weight osmotic agent that induces a colloid osmotic pressure gradient. This makes it very attractive for long dialysis dwells, especially in patients with ultrafiltration failure associated with fast transport rates of low-molecular-weight solutes. A drawback of both amino acids and icodextrin is that they should only be applied once daily. Biocompatible solutions can be used for all exchanges, but a number of advantages ascribed are not very relevant. Their main advantages are the absence of inflow pain and probably the reduction in the formation of interstitial fibrotic alterations, which may be protective against the development of encapsulating peritoneal sclerosis.

Suggested Reading

Davies SJ, Woodrow G, Donovan K, Plum J, Williams P, Johansson AC, et al:
Icodextrin improves the fluid status of peritoneal dialysis patients: results of a
double-blind randomized controlled trial.
J Am Soc Nephrol 2003;14:2338–2344.

Del Peso G, Jimenez-Heffernan JA, Selgas R, Remon C, Ossorio M, et al:
Biocompatible dialysis solutions preserve mesothelial cell and vessel wall
integrity. A case-control study on human biopsies.
Perit Dial Int 2016;36:129–134.

Fan SLS, Pile T, Punzalan S, Raftery MJ, Yaqoob MM:
Randomized controlled study of biocompatible peritoneal dialysis solutions:
effects on residual renal function.
Kidney Int 2008;73:200–206.

Garcia-Lopez E, Lindholm B, Davies S:
An update on peritoneal dialysis solutions.
Nat Rev Nephrol 2012;8:224–233.

Ho-dac-Pannekeet MM, Schouten N, Langedijk MJ, Hiralall JK,
de Waart DW, Struijk DG, Krediet RT:
Peritoneal transport characteristics with glucose polymer dialysate.
Kidney Int 1996;50:979–968.

Johnson DW, Brown FG, Clarke M, Boudville N, Elias TJ, Foo MWY, et al:
The effect of low glucose degradation product, neutral pH versus standard
peritoneal dialysis solutions on peritoneal membrane function:
the balAZN trial.
Nephrol Dial Transplant 2012;27:4445–4453.

Jones MR, Gehr TW, Burkart JW, Hamburger RJ, Kraus AP Jr, et al:
Replacement of amino acid and protein losses
with 1.1% amino acid peritoneal dialysis solution.
Perit Dial Int 1998;18:210–216.

Kawanishi K, Honda K, Tsukada M, Oda H, Nitta K:
Neutral solution low in glucose degradation products is associated
with less peritoneal fibrosis and vascular sclerosis in patients receiving
peritoneal dialysis.
Perit Dial Int 2013;33:242–251.

Krediet RT:
The physiology of peritoneal solute, water, and lymphatic transport;
in: Nolph and Gokal's Textbook of Peritoneal Dialysis, ed 3.
Berlin, Springer, 2009, pp 137–172.

Mistry CD, Gokal R, Peers E:
A randomized multicenter clinical trial comparing isosmolar icodextrin
with hyperosmolar glucose solutions in CAPD. Midas Study Group.
Kidney Int 1994;46:496–503.

Rippe B, Simonsen O, Heimburger O, Christensson A, Haraldsson B,
Stelin G, et al:
Long-term clinical effects of a peritoneal dialysis fluid with less glucose
degradation products.
Kidney Int 2001;59:348–357.

Srivastava S, Hildebrand S, Fan SLS:
Long-term follow-up of patients randomized to biocompatible or
conventional peritoneal dialysis solutions show no difference in peritonitis
or technique survival.
Kidney Int 2011;80:986–991.

Tjong HL, Swart R, van den Berg JW, Fieren MW:
Amino acid-based peritoneal dialysis solution: new perspectives.
Perit Dial Int 2009;29:384–393.

Tjong HL, van den Berg JW, Waltimena JL, Rietveld T, van Dijk LJ,
van der Wiel AM, et al:
Dialysate as food: combined amino acids and glucose dialysate improves protein
anabolism in renal failure patients on automated peritoneal dialysis.
J Am Soc Nephrol 2005;16:1486–1493.

Vardhan A, Zweers MM, Gokal R, Krediet RT:
A solutions portfolio approach in peritoneal dialysis.
Kidney Int 2003;88:S114-S123.

Wieslander AP, Nordin MK, Kjellstrand PT, Boberg UC:
Toxicity of peritoneal dialysis fluids on cultured fibroblasts, L-929.
Kidney Int 1991;39:55–58.

Chapter 9

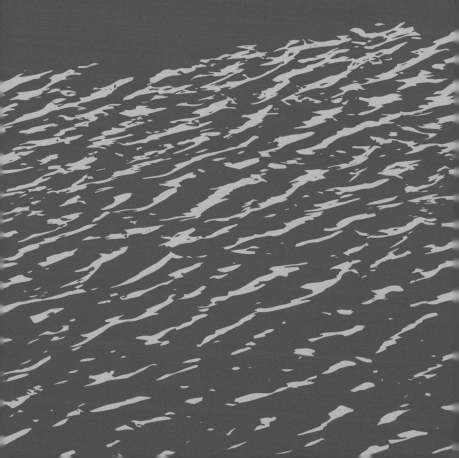

Chapter 10

Long-Term Peritoneal Dialysis and Encapsulating Peritoneal Sclerosis

Long-Term Peritoneal Dialysis and Encapsulating Peritoneal Sclerosis

Long-term use of the peritoneum as a dialysis membrane can lead to its abrasion, characterized by both anatomic and functional changes. Knowledge on the morphological alterations stems from autopsy material and peritoneal biopsies that were never taken at predefined time intervals, but always occasionally. No prospective study is available on serial peritoneal biopsies, which renders analysis of their prevalence, sequence, severity, and precise relationships with peritoneal function parameters impossible. Keeping this in mind, a number of alterations in peritoneal tissues may be important.

The number of mesothelial cells is lower in patients on long-term PD than in those starting PD. Also, acute peritonitis is associated with a temporary loss of mesothelial cells. The mesothelial-to-mesenchymal transition (MMT) has been described as an event that can occur during the first 2 years of treatment. In this process, mesothelial cells are transformed into myofibroblasts. Functionally, this phenomenon is associated with high effluent concentrations of cancer antigen (CA)-125, vascular endothelial growth factor (VEGF), and fast peritoneal transport of small solutes. These biomarker and functional changes disappear spontaneously, suggesting that MMT is a temporary event. It has been suggested that matrix metalloproteins could be the triggers of long-term morphological alterations, but no serial histology is available to support this claim. The distance between 2 adjacent mesothelial cells exceeds 500 Å and, combined with functional data, excludes a barrier function to peritoneal solute transport. However, vasoactive substances released by mesothelial cells like VEGF may influence peritoneal transport.

The number of peritoneal microvessels can increase after 2–3 years of PD, which is accompanied by increased transport rates of small solutes and decreased ultrafiltration. These are accompanied by high effluent VEGF concentrations, similar to diabetic microvasculopathy. The vessels show diabetiform changes on electron microscopy, e.g., duplications of their basement membrane. Subendothelial hyalinosis of both arteries and venules sometimes leading to luminal obliteration is the hallmark of the vasculopathy on light microscopy. It is likely that the degree of vasculopathy will increase with the time on PD, but this is unlikely for the number of vessels. The latter is reflected in parameters of small solute transport; assessment of the severity of vasculopathy requires tissue examination.

Peritoneal interstitial tissue is composed of an extracellular matrix consisting of proteoglycans and hyaluronan. The latter is a hydrophilic glycosaminoglycan not bound to a core protein. The interstitium also contains blood and lymphatic vessels, some collagen fibers, and deposed advanced glycosylation end products, the latter already 6 months after the start of PD. Fibrotic alterations can develop submesothelially in the parietal peritoneum but also more generalized. The fibers consist mainly of collagen-1. The thickness of the parietal submesothelial compact zone has been studied in most detail, although encapsulating peritoneal sclerosis (EPS) is especially a disease of the visceral peritoneum. Submesothelial thickness is not only determined by the amount of fibrotic tissue but also by its hydration state. Also, ultrasonographically, there is no difference in peritoneal thickness between patients treated for <1 year compared to those on long-term PD. These data suggest that the importance of submesothelial thickness is overrated and not inevitably present in every long-term PD patient.

Encapsulating Peritoneal Sclerosis

EPS is the most serious complication of long-term PD. It occurs in 2% of patients starting PD and in 4% of those treated >2 years. Patients with EPS have thickening of the bowel walls, mesentery, and/ or parietal peritoneum. The bowel loops are adherent and covered by thick fibrous tissue, often adherent to the abdominal wall. Clinically, EPS is characterized by signs and symptoms of bowel obstruction that may be intermittent initially. The subsequent development of malnutrition is the major cause of death, apart from postoperative complications. EPS can also occur after kidney transplantation. Besides long-term exposure to dialysis solutions, other factors may also be involved in the excessive fibrotic response, e.g., an inflammatory reaction, like T-helper lymphocytes and various growth factors. Medical treatment should be aimed at avoiding malnutrition and often requires parenteral nutrition. Favorable effects have also been ascribed to corticosteroids and tamoxifen. Surgical treatment including peritonectomy and enterolysis requires specialized surgeons and is not possible everywhere.

Peritoneal Transport

Diffusion rates of low-molecular-weight solutes like creatinine and glucose may start to increase after about 2 years. This is likely caused by glucose-induced neoangiogenesis leading to a larger number of perfused peritoneal microvessels available for solute transport: the effective peritoneal surface area. The faster transport rate of glucose leads to a faster disappearance of the crystalloid osmotic gradient and thereby reduced transcapillary ultrafiltration. The larger number of perfused microvessels in itself means that more pores are available for fluid transport, but this effect is counteracted by the increased disappearance of the osmotic gradient. It has turned out that the larger number of pores is associated with higher transport rates of small-pore fluid transport, while a reduced osmotic pressure gradient is related to a lower rate of free water transport (FWT). Net ultrafiltration (the sum of small-pore fluid transport, FWT, and lymphatic absorption) is lower in patients with a large effective peritoneal surface area.

The development of an increased effective surface area not only involves small-pore transport of low-molecular-weight solutes but also the transport of serum proteins from the circulation to peritoneal dialysate. Small proteins like β_2-microglobulin are transported through the small interendothelial pores, but from albumin onwards serum proteins can only be transported through sparse, large interendothelial pores. In contrast to low-molecular-weight solutes, the transport of macromolecules is not only determined by their diffusion coefficient but also size-selectively hindered either by the average size of the large pores or by properties of the interstitium. This intrinsic permeability of the peritoneal membrane to macromolecules can be expressed as the restriction coefficient. This parameter is the slope of the linear regression that is present between peritoneal clearances of selected serum proteins and their molecular weight, when plotted on a double logarithmic scale. This representation of the size-selective peritoneal barrier to macromolecular transport increases during the follow-up of patients. The precise meaning of this phenomenon is unknown, but it likely represents interstitial changes.

Fluid transport in long-term PD has already been discussed in Chapter 1 Anatomy and Physiology of the Peritoneum. Not only high solute transport rates are important in the pathogenesis of ultrafiltration failure but also impaired FWT. The latter is likely explained by binding of water to interstitial collagen. Severely reduced FWT is the strongest predictor of EPS, and its determination should be included in the long-term follow-up of PD patients.

Suggested Reading

Coester AM, Smit W, Struijk DG, Parikova A, Krediet RT:
Longitudinal analysis of fluid transport and their determinants in PD patients.
Perit Dial Int 2014;34:195–203.

Honda K, Nitta K, Horita S, Yumura W, Nihei H:
Morphological changes in the peritoneal vasculature of patients on CAPD with ultrafiltration failure.
Nephron 1996;72:171–176.

Krediet RT, Lopes Barreto D, Struijk DG:
Can free water transport be used as a clinical parameter for peritoneal fibrosis in long-term PD patients?
Perit Dial Int 2016;36:124–128.

Krediet RT, Struijk DG:
Peritoneal changes in patients on long-term peritoneal dialysis.
Nat Rev Nephrol 2013;9:419–429.

Morelle J, Sow A, Houtem H, Bouzin C, Crott R, Devuyst O, Goffin E:
Interstitial fibrosis restricts osmotic water transport in encapsulating peritoneal sclerosis.
J Am Soc Nephrol 2015;26:1521–1533.

Sampimon DE, Coester AM, Struijk DG, Krediet RT:
The time course of peritoneal transport parameters in peritoneal dialysis patients who develop encapsulating peritoneal sclerosis.
Nephrol Dial Transplant 2011;26:291–298.

Tranu T, Florea L, Paduraru D, Georgescu SO, Francu LL, Stan CI:
Morphological changes of the peritoneal membrane in patients with long-term dialysis.
Rom J Morphol Embryol 2014;55:927–932.

Van Esch S, Struijk DG, Krediet RT:
The natural time-course of membrane alterations during peritoneal
dialysis is partly altered by peritonitis.
Perit Dial Int 2016;36:448–456.

Williams JD, Craig KJ, Topley N, et al:
Morphologic changes in the peritoneal membrane of patients with renal disease.
J Am Soc Nephrol 2002;13:470–479.

Yanez-Mo M, Lara-Pezzi E, Selgas R, et al:
Peritoneal dialysis and epithelial-to-mesenchymal transition of mesothelial cells.
N Engl J Med 2003;348:403–413.